1984

Planning Hospital Health Promotion Services for Business and Industry

AHA_{SM}

American Hospital Publishing, Inc.,
a wholly owned subsidiary
of the American Hospital Association

Library of Congress Cataloging in Publication Data

Bader, Barry S.
  Planning hospital health promotion services for business and industry.

    Written by Barry S. Bader, Lynn Dickey Jones, and
Sharon Yenney.
    Based on a series of conferences conducted by the
American Hospital Association starting in November 1979.
    "AHA catalog no. 070175"—P.
    Bibliography: p.
    1. Hospitals—Health promotion services—Congresses.
2. Occupational health services—Congresses.   I. Jones,
Lynn Dickey.   II. Yenney, Sharon.   III. American Hospital
Association.   IV. Title.
RA975.5.H4B33   1984   362.1'7   84-16848
ISBN 0-939450-36-4

AHA catalog no. 070175

Printed in the U.S.A.
2M-10/82-2-0643
1.2M-9/84-0047

Contents

Preface. v
Acknowledgments. vii
Introduction. 1
Chapter 1.   Health Promotion Services. 5
Chapter 2.   Hospital's Perspective. 17
Chapter 3.   Employer's Perspective. 23
Chapter 4.   Market-Oriented Approach to Planning. 29
Chapter 5.   Impact on Hospital and Business Environment. 57
Chapter 6.   Six Success Stories. 65
Appendix A.   Survey of Conference Participants. 85
Appendix B.   Corporate Structures for Health Promotion Activities. . 93
Bibliography 105

Preface

The content of this book, *Planning Hospital Health Promotion Services for Business and Industry,* is based on an American Hospital Association conference entitled "New Business Opportunities for Hospitals: Health Promotion Services for Local Industry," which was developed in response to hospitals' requests for guidance in planning employee health promotion programs for business and industry. The purpose of the conference was to provide hospital decision makers with a framework for developing financially viable health promotion programs to meet the present and future needs of business and industry. The conference was designed by marketing experts and emphasized case study presentations by hospitals that have actual experience in implementing programs for industry.

The conference was initially conducted in November 1979. However, because of continuing interest and requests from the field, the conference was repeated four times during the following three years. This book was developed as a result of the consistently growing demand from hospitals for information and guidelines on planning programs for business and industry. The book focuses on:

- The current economic and social developments that are affecting industry and creating new business opportunities for hospitals
- A review of the types of programs available and examples of several hospitals that are at present marketing health promotion services
- The importance of conducting a thorough assessment of both the health promotion needs of industry and the hospital's internal resources and capabilities to provide services
- The marketing concepts needed to plan health promotion programs and services for business and industry

Acknowledgments

This book was written by Barry S. Bader, Bader & Associates, Kensington, Maryland; Lynn Dickey Jones, employee health education manager, Center for Health Promotion, American Hospital Association; and Sharon Yenney, director of health promotion, Parkside Medical Services, Chicago, and was based on the content of the conference "New Business Opportunities for Hospitals: Health Promotion Services for Local Industry."

A special debt of thanks must go to Robert Rotanz of Rotanz Associates, Berkeley, New Jersey, and Ruth Behrens, former director, Center for Health Promotion, American Hospital Association, for developing the conference on which this book is based.

The development of the book is largely the result of the valuable ideas and information of the following dedicated health care professionals who shared their expertise and experiences by participating in the conference and contributing to the book: Paula Bills, manager, Priority Systems, Overlook Hospital, Summit, New Jersey; Linda Hawes Clever, M.D., chairman, Department of Occupational Health, Presbyterian Hospital of Pacific Medical Center, San Francisco; Michael J. Gallagher, vice-president of operations, Swedish American Hospital, Rockford, Illinois; Stephen Gelineau, assistant administrator, Union Hospital, Lynn, Massachusetts; Willis B. Goldbeck, director, Washington Business Group on Health, Washington, DC; David J. Heritage, director, Occupational Health Service, Franklin County Hospital, Greenfield, Massachusetts; and Donald W. Zeigler, director, Good Health Program, Skokie Valley Community Hospital, Skokie, Illinois.

The "Selected Resources for Developing Employee Health Programs in Occupational Settings" was compiled for the Center for Health Promotion of the American Hospital Association by Katherine M. Huff, health education evaluation consultant, Chicago. Additional updating of this list was completed by Mary Woodrow, R.N., director, Health Education Services, El Camino Hospital, Mountain View, California, and Lynn Dickey Jones.

The book was edited by Sandra L. Weiss, staff editor, under the supervision of Marjorie E. Weissman, manager, Book Department, American Hospital Association.

Introduction

This publication provides key hospital decision makers with a framework for making sound judgments and decisions about developing health promotion programs for business and industry. The book is designed to facilitate the development of effective, salable programs that deliver what they promise, make good use of hospital resources, and meet the needs of prospective business and industry clients. Following are highlights of each chapter to help the reader gain a sense of the range of information and topics covered.

Chapter 1 classifies the types of services that hospitals currently are providing to business and industry into three categories (employee assistance programs; wellness, or life-style, programs; and occupational health programs) and provides data about the effectiveness of each type of program at the work site. This information is of special interest because the amount of data on the effectiveness of health promotion programs in business and industry varies considerably. Although numerous examples exist to demonstrate that employee assistance programs provide a significant payback to the employer, little documentation is available on the effectiveness of occupational health programs because these services are most often government-mandated to protect employees' health and safety. Similarly, data concerning the effectiveness of content areas within wellness and life-style programs varies. Because many future clients will undoubtedly demand evidence that health promotion programs produce benefits for employers, no hospital should undertake any program without first being aware of the available cost-effectiveness information for each program area as documented both by research and by data collected within individual work settings.

Chapter 2 looks at the provision of health promotion services from the hospital's perspective. The hospital decision maker must assess the hospital's overall goals and objectives for health promotion before actual planning begins. This assessment process includes examining the hospital's mission; identifying and ranking the potential benefits of health promotion services for the hospital, the consumer, and local business and industry; and surveying the local business market to determine whether it is ready for a new product such as health promotion services. Unless these issues are addressed during the preliminary planning stage, valuable time and energy may be spent developing a product that does not fit with the hospital's overall mission, does not provide desired benefits to all groups involved, or is not readily acceptable to business and industry.

Chapter 3 examines the provision of health promotion services from the employer's perspective. The chapter describes a business representative's list of the six most common types of employer programs and identifies some of the considerations that are important to employers who might be potential clients for a hospital's health promotion services.

Chapter 4 provides a process for planning health promotion services that uses many of the basic elements of a marketing strategy. The process, which consists of six steps, can be divided into a research and analysis phase and an action planning phase. The six steps are general assessment, market orientation, industry assessment, hospital assessment, building a program, and planning for sales. The first four steps form the research and analysis phase, and the last two are the action planning phase. At the end of each step, there are questions that a key hospital decision maker responsible for the program should answer before proceeding to the next development phase. Although these steps are presented in consecutive order, many of these steps overlap during the actual planning process. It is vitally important to recognize that none of the steps can be overlooked and no elements within each individual step can be bypassed if the institution is to proceed smoothly from planning to implementation.

Chapter 5 describes the impact of health promotion on the hospital and business environment. This chapter is based on the actual experiences of hospitals that have already developed and implemented programs. It describes what is likely to happen within the hospital, at the work site, and to the individual who administers or manages the program as a result of instituting the health promotion program. It also suggests actions that can be taken to prevent some problems from occurring and to overcome some of the resistance to new programs. The hospital manager or decision maker who is prepared for these potential problems or reactions is in a much stronger position to ensure smooth, successful program implementation.

Chapter 6 highlights six hospitals that have successfully developed and implemented health promotion programs for local business and industry. These brief summaries describe the hospital, its service area, program objectives, and components and provide some details about program development, such as funding, fee structures, and marketing strategies. Also, the program manager from each hospital offers some suggestions for success based on his or her own experience.

Appendix A provides the most up-to-date summary available about what hospitals actually are doing in providing health promotion services for business and industry. Participants in a series of American Hospital Association conferences, which were the basis of this publication, were surveyed to find out what types of programs hospitals have developed, whether market research has been conducted, where programs are located and how they are staffed within the hospital, the amount of time required to sell a program, the amount of start-up money allocated for program development, the pricing strategy, and the most common problems encountered in program development and implementation. Although the survey does not provide definitive information about how a specific hospital should develop a program, it does offer insights into how 150 hospitals have operated.

Appendix B offers an attorney's expert opinion on why hospitals should consider developing a separate corporate structure for a successful and profitable health promotion program. This material is for attorneys rather than laypersons, and it is therefore suggested that an attorney be involved early in the planning process to determine whether or not a separate corporate structure should be considered.

Finally, an annotated bibliography provides a basic set of readings about health promotion in the work place. Included in the bibliography is some of the most important literature on background studies of health promotion in the work place, planning and developing programs, and costs and benefits of health promotion in the work place as well as content-specific literature dealing with alcoholism and drug abuse, hypertension, nutrition and weight control, physical fitness, risk assessment, screening programs, smoking cessation, and stress management. There is also a list of additional general readings. The bibliography is not designed to be an all-inclusive survey of the literature. While it is unlikely that anyone will have either the time or energy to become familiar with all these references, it is vitally important that key hospital decision makers and program implementers have a good grasp of the literature that supports as well as provides cautions about health promotion programs for business and industry. Without this background, program planners may be unable to answer some of the important questions posed by business and industry about the effectiveness of health promotion programs.

Chapter 1

Health Promotion Services

The promotion of good health is hardly a new idea. The scourges of overeating, tobacco, and alcohol abuse were first proclaimed, not by the *New England Journal of Medicine,* but by others long before that august journal began publishing. Back in 166 B.C. the Roman playwright Terence wrote, "When we are well, we all have good advice for those who are ill" (ref. 1). In 1665 someone must have been extolling good health behavior to lead the French writer Francois La Rochefoucauld to write in his book of *Maxims:* "Preserving the health by too severe a rule is a wearisome malady" (ref. 1).

Health Promotion Defined

The simplest definition of health promotion is the promotion of health. However, for the purposes of this book, the definition adopted by the American Hospital Association is used. In its 1979 policy document *The Hospital's Responsibility for Health Promotion,* the AHA defined *health promotion* this way: "Health promotion (including health information and health education) is the process of fostering awareness, influencing attitudes, and identifying alternatives so that individuals can make informed choices and change their behavior in order to achieve an optimum level of physical and mental health and improve their physical and social environment" (ref. 2).

Health promotion differs from the provision of traditional medical care in that it is a *process* rather than a specific therapy or treatment and it requires individuals to take personal responsibility for their health behavior. Individuals are active participants in their own health care rather than passive recipients dependent on medical professionals to provide specific treatment. Health promotion takes a comprehensive and holistic approach to caring for the total person. It goes beyond the detection or treatment of physical illness or symptoms to encompass the mental and spiritual as well as physical aspects of health.

This distinction between health promotion and medical care is further delineated in the 1979 Surgeon General's report on health promotion and disease prevention, which states (ref. 3):

Medical care begins with the sick and seeks to keep them alive, make them well, or minimize their disability.

Disease prevention begins with a threat to health—a disease or environmental hazard—and seeks to protect as many people as possible from the harmful consequences that threaten.

Health promotion begins with people who are basically healthy and seeks the development of community and individual measures which can help them to develop life-styles that can maintain and enhance the state of well-being.

Types of Health Promotion Programs

Hospitals are directing their health promotion efforts to three primary audiences: patients, employees, and the community. Hospital-based programs for patients are aimed at helping them manage their illnesses and get well. Programs directed at the hospital's own employees, members of the community, and employees of local businesses are aimed at apparently healthy nonpatients and focus on helping them stay well and achieve optimum levels of health. This book concentrates on three types of health promotion services that are likely to be of greatest interest to local industry. These are employee assistance programs; occupational health programs; and wellness, or life-style, programs.

Employee Assistance Programs

An employee assistance program is designed to help businesses provide assistance to employees who have personal problems that are adversely affecting the employee's physical, psychological, or emotional health and are consequently interfering with the employee's job performance. Such problems may involve alcohol or drug abuse, family or marital problems, or financial or legal difficulties.

Employee assistance programs focus on early problem identification and referral to appropriate counseling or therapy before a crisis occurs. An employee assistance program is designed to offer confidential and professional assistance to any employee in a stressful situation, either personal or work related, before it becomes necessary to terminate the employee because of declining job performance.

A hospital may provide the following services to employers who want to set up an employee assistance program:

- Consultation with top management in designing an organizational policy
- Training programs to help supervisors learn how to identify and refer for professional counseling and diagnosis those employees who have performance problems that do not respond to supervisory techniques
- Training for an in-house staff member who will act as a referral counselor to coordinate arrangements with appropriate outside agencies that will provide counseling or treatment for an employee's specific problem
- Assistance in identifying referral resources, such as agencies within the community that will provide consultation and treatment for the employee's problem
- Treatment for alcohol or drug-related problems
- Record keeping and evaluation of the effectiveness of the program

Employee assistance programs may rely on referrals by the supervisor or self-referrals by employees. Because it is recognized that many personal problems can be successfully resolved if they are handled at an early stage, employees are encouraged to use the program services voluntarily. However, if a supervisor observes that an employee's job performance is declining because of personal problems, the supervisor is encouraged to refer the employee to the program rather than trying to discuss or diagnose the personal problem with the employee. This enables supervisors to use their time more productively by limiting their involvement to managing the employee's work performance.

The most crucial aspect of an effective employee assistance program is maintaining confidentiality concerning all employees involved in the program. A hospital providing this type of service to a business has a major advantage in this regard because, as an outside agency, the hospital can maintain information about an employee using the program without jeopardizing that employee's position on the job.

Wellness, or Life-Style, Programs

Wellness, or life-style, programs are designed to help businesses keep their employees well. Hospitals can provide resources to help employers create a supportive environment at the work place that encourages employees to take personal responsibility for their own health. Wellness programs are aimed at helping employees change life-style habits that may increase their health risks. These programs are directed at helping employees make such changes in their life-styles as reducing stress, increasing exercise, or improving their diets. Wellness programs can cover a broad spectrum of activities, such as:

- Health hazard appraisals or assessments, which are screening programs to identify a person's health risks before illness or symptoms of disease occur and to assess an individual's future prospects for good or ill health. Health hazard appraisals and projections are based on quantitative data about an individual's personal and family health history and present life-style behaviors and habits and may also include actual physical measurements and clinical test results.

- Screening for symptoms of specific health problems, such as hypertension, diabetes, and glaucoma.
- Health education classes and informational seminars directed at educating, motivating, and changing individuals' health behavior to reduce health risks in a variety of areas, such as smoking cessation, stress management, weight control, and nutrition.
- Physical fitness evaluations and aerobic exercise programs.
- Activities designed to increase employee awareness and involvement in healthy behaviors at the work place. These activities might include promoting walk-to-work and stair-climbing campaigns; sponsoring discounted corporate memberships in fitness clubs; establishing designated no-smoking sections in employee work areas; offering healthy low-fat menu selections in the employee cafeteria; and introducing other company-sponsored incentives, such as awards and certificates, T-shirts, buttons, or paid "wellness" days to encourage and reward employees' involvement in healthy activities.

Occupational Health Programs

Occupational health programs are designed to protect the physical health and safety of employees at the work place and to prevent work-related illness and injury. Because many businesses do not have the volume of employees necessary to justify setting up an in-house medical department to conduct occupational health programs, they may come to depend on local community hospitals to provide the necessary medical personnel and expertise as well as specialized screening and testing services and facilities to help them create a safe and healthy work environment for their employees. Occupational health services focus on assessing the work environment for possible health hazards, physically screening individuals for any health problems related to their specific job function in order to protect against injury, and educating employees on how to prevent work-related illness or injury. Other occupational health services also performed by hospitals include diagnosing and providing emergency care for work-related accidents and injuries, conducting disability evaluations, and processing workers' compensation claims.

Occupational health programs cover a broad range of preventive testing and educational services, such as:

- Preemployment, preplacement, executive, or return-to-work physical examinations tailored to the employee's job

- Identification of hazardous or toxic substances at the work site and development of worker safety and protection programs
- Medical surveillance of individuals exposed to dangerous substances at the work place
- Audiometric testing and hearing conservation services to teach workers how to prevent ear injuries
- Back care programs and educational seminars on how to prevent injury through exercise programs and proper lifting techniques
- Rehabilitation services to return employees to work as soon as possible after injury
- Consultation on compliance with regulations of the Occupational Safety and Health Administration (OSHA)

Program Effectiveness

By entering the health promotion market, not-for-profit hospitals are entering a field already identified as a fertile marketplace by the private sector. Reputable exercise clubs, weight control programs, and smoking cessation clinics have become million dollar industries. In the United States, there are a reported 3,000 gymnasiums, figure salons, and luxury health spas that gross about $400 million a year in membership fees alone (ref. 4). According to one estimate, Americans spend $10 billion annually on weight reduction alone (ref. 5). The best-known weight control clinic, Weight Watchers International, reports gross revenues in excess of $15 million and profits of more than $1 million (ref. 6).

However, all this marketplace activity cannot minimize the need to ask some fundamental questions: Does health promotion work? Does it motivate individuals to change their health behavior? Does it help individuals live longer, healthier lives? Does it improve employee morale? Does it result in increased worker productivity and decreased absenteeism and job-related injuries? Does it reduce the costs of acute medical care?

These questions are important. Physicians and other health care professionals will pose them as a hospital gears up to provide health promotion services to businesses. Employers will pose them to the hospital seeking to market health promotion services.

Although all the evidence is not in, the following examples discussed under the types of health promotion programs indicate that properly planned health promotion activities have the potential to motivate health behavior changes, decrease worker absenteeism and job-related injuries, improve productivity, and eventually reduce some medical care costs. In addition, involvement in health promotion activities in some cases appears to improve morale and is perceived by participants as improving the quality of their lives.

Data on the effectiveness of health promotion programs at the work site are beginning to appear in the literature. Briefly, here are some of the positive reports about the effectiveness of health promotion:

Employee Assistance Programs

Employee assistance programs focus on improving employees' on-the-job performance by offering confidential counseling and treatment for a wide range of personal problems. Current estimates are that 10 percent of all employees have serious personal problems; 25 percent of productivity is lost at all ages, but more from ages 30 to 49; 50 percent of employees' personal problems are alcohol related; and the use of health insurance by alcoholics is three times that of nonalcoholics (p. 28 of ref. 7).

Alcoholism accounts for an estimated cost to industry of $25 billion to $40 billion each year (ref. 8). Alcoholic employees are absent 2-1/2 times as often and have an accident rate 3.6 times greater than nonalcoholic workers (ref. 9). North American Rockwell estimated a loss of $50,000 per alcoholic worker, and the United California Bank of Los Angeles estimated that in a 10,000-person work force, alcoholic employees would cost the firm $1 million (ref. 9). Drug abusers also have been shown to have high rates of absenteeism and job-related injuries (ref. 9). To a lesser extent, employees with emotional, marital, legal, or financial problems also have problems performing adequately on the job.

To combat these statistics, some companies have set up employee assistance programs. Following are selected examples of such companies:

- Illinois Bell Telephone has had an alcohol rehabilitation program since 1951. A study of 650 employees in the program showed an estimated direct savings of $459,000 in reduced absences resulting from sickness. Some 58 percent, of the participants were rated "good performers" after the program, compared with 22 percent before. "Poor performance" ratings dropped from 28 to 12 percent (ref. 9).
- E. I. du Pont de Nemours & Co., a pioneer in alcohol abuse programs since 1942, spends an average of $1,342.50 for each of 176 new alcoholic patients under treatment each year. However, du Pont estimates that it saves $419,200 a year from decreased absenteeism, because alcoholic employees average 13 disability days per year, compared with 5.8 for a control group (ref. 9).
- Kimberly Clark employees participating in an employee assistance program had a 70 percent reduction in accidents for the year after participation compared with the year before (ref. 8).
- General Motors reports that 44,000 employees at more than 180 sites have used its employee assistance program. This is 7 percent of the company's total employees in North America. General Motors estimates that 10 percent of its employees have severe personal problems. Dur-

ing the first year after the company began the program, costs resulting from lost time decreased 40 percent, sickness and accident benefits decreased 60 percent, grievances decreased 50 percent, and on-the-job accidents decreased 50 percent. General Motors estimates at least a 3 to 1 return on dollars invested in its employee assistance program (p. 29 of ref. 7).

- Equitable Life Assurance Society indicated a 5.52 to 1 return on dollars invested in its employee assistance program (p. 29 of ref. 7).
- Kennecott Copper Corporation of Salt Lake City reports that its Insight Program of confidential counseling and referral has helped more than 9,000 employees since 1970 and returned $6 for every $1 invested in the program. In a study of 150 employees, absenteeism was reduced 53 percent; sickness and accident costs dropped by 75 percent; and health, medical, and surgical costs were cut by 55 percent (ref. 9).
- Group Health Association, a Washington, DC, health maintenance organization, reports that users of mental health counseling benefits reduced their nonpsychiatric physician visits by 30.7 percent and their use of laboratory and x-ray services by 29.8 percent (ref. 8).

Wellness, or Life-Style, Programs

Poor health habits are costly. The leading causes of death today are heart disease (48.4 percent of total deaths), cancer (20.6 percent), and accidents (5.5 percent). They account for almost 75 percent of total deaths (p. 28 of ref. 7). These causes of death have been associated with a number of health risk factors that are life-style related, such as smoking, overweight, dietary fat intake, and lack of exercise. A combination of improper eating, overeating, and lack of exercise leads to greater risk or aggravation of cardiovascular illness, diabetes, hernia, and gall bladder disease.

Life-style, or wellness, programs aim at educating and motivating the individual to reduce health risks by participating in a variety of health promotion activities, such as exercise or smoking cessation classes. If employees can reduce their own risks, then in the process of improving their health, they may also help to reduce the employer's overall health care costs.

For example, in the area of smoking, it is the employer who bears most of the costs associated with smoking-related illnesses. For many years, the National Center for Health Statistics has gathered data on cigarette smokers. This survey has consistently found that smokers are ill more often than nonsmokers, lose more days from work, and are more likely to suffer from chronic conditions that limit activity. From these surveys it has been calculated that each year an excess of nearly 150 million sick days are the result of the extra amounts of illness experienced by cigarette smokers (ref. 10).

The Advisory Council on Education for Health reports that employee cigarette smoking cost an estimated $36 billion in lost productivity during 1980 (ref. 11). A 1979 report on the economics of employee smoking, prepared by Action on Smoking and Health, cited the following (ref. 12):

- One-fifth of all lost workdays in the United States are attributable to the effects of cigarette smoking.
- A two-pack-a-day smoker is absent from work 150 percent more than a nonsmoker.
- Medical and disability payments and insurance costs are greatly increased as a result of the smoking habit.
- Lost production time as a result of handling smoking paraphernalia and the problem of smoking in hazardous work areas indicate that the reduction of smoking in the work area is a significant factor in saving money and increasing efficiency for almost any business operation.

The potential annual savings to industry per employee who stops smoking has been calculated by the American Health Foundation as $345 by the end of the first three years of nonsmoking and an additional $224 per year per employee after 3 to 10 years (ref. 13).

Following are some examples of companies that have set up wellness, or life-style, programs:

- Speedcall Corporation, a small communications manufacturing firm in California, has implemented an effective smoking cessation program for its employees that has resulted in decreased smoking-related illnesses and absenteeism. The company president believes that recent increases in productivity and reductions in employee health care costs are, in part, caused by the smoking cessation program (ref. 14).
- Dow Chemical's smoking cessation program participants have maintained a 70 percent success rate a full year following the program (ref. 8).
- Campbell Soup Company found a cessation rate of 25 percent at the end of the year among 70 employees who participated in a company-sponsored smoking cessation clinic. In addition, Campbell conducts an employee cardiovascular risk factor screening program that includes both physical and laboratory evaluations. Hypertension control programs have evaluated 10,000 employees since 1968, with in-house treatment programs being undertaken to reduce costs. A screening program for colon and rectal cancer has saved the company $245,000 in direct insurance payments and absenteeism costs (ref. 7).
- Ford Motor Company has a cardiovascular risk intervention program. The company found that although heart attacks accounted for only 1.5 percent of employee health problems, they accounted for 29 percent of the total health care costs at Ford's Michigan headquarters. The Ford program identifies high-risk employees and offers such assistance as

smoking cessation clinics, cardiovascular exercise programs, and healthful menus in the cafeteria. Ford also encourages employees to participate in stress management programs offered in the community (ref. 15).

- The National Aeronautics and Space Administration (NASA) reports a 52 percent improvement in job performance as a result of a fitness program for employees at its Washington, DC, headquarters (ref. 8). Participants reported more positive work attitudes and less strain and tension at their jobs.
- When a Goodyear plant in Norkjoping, Sweden, introduced an employee fitness program, absenteeism by participants fell by nearly one-half (ref. 16).
- Physicians at Cornell Medical Center have analyzed the costs of treating hypertensive workers who are members of the United Storeworkers Union in New York City at their work site. Cornell's analysis shows that controlling hypertension among affected workers appears to be cost-effective (ref. 3).
- New York Telephone, Burlington Industries of Greensboro, North Carolina, and American Telephone and Telegraph have reported good results from their hypertension screening programs. New York Telephone has developed a multiphasic screening program that includes blood pressure screening, referral, and follow-up for all employees. More than 10 percent of the screened employees were found to have elevated blood pressure, and of these employees, half had their condition subsequently brought under control. Estimated annual savings from reduced absenteeism alone at one site were about $30,000 (ref. 16).

Occupational Health Programs

The federal government estimates that 14,000 job-related deaths and millions of disabling injuries occur every year (ref. 17). Some experts would add as many as 25 million unreported injuries per year, with 390,000 cases of work-related disease resulting in about 100,000 deaths annually (ref. 17). Accidents are the fourth leading cause of death in the United States, and 50 percent of disabling injuries occur on the job (ref. 9).

Structuring the work environment so that it is safe is likely to produce the most significant reductions in accidents and long-term illnesses. Many businesses, such as the Gilette Company, Caterpillar Tractor Company, and General Motors Corporation, conduct aggressive safety and accident prevention programs and preplacement and periodic testing in an effort to prevent injuries, costly hospitalization, and lost work time. For example, low back pain and injury are responsible for much lost work time each year. Workers' compensation for low back pain costs employers some $250 million a year (ref. 8). Some companies have developed screening criteria to prevent employees susceptible to back injury from working in areas where back injury is likely to occur (ref. 19). Because of the cost to industry and the employee, many businesses also provide training in safe lifting and handling techniques to help reduce back injury.

Although little comprehensive cost-effectiveness data exist for occupational health services, the federal Occupational Safety and Health Act (OSHA) and the Toxic Substances Control Act mandate that business and industry assume responsibility to protect the health and safety of their employees. These regulations, as well as businesses' own interest in the health of their employees, offer the most significant stimulus for business and industry to provide services for the safety and prevention of occupational disease and illness at the work place.

Potential of Health Promotion Programs

It appears that properly managed health promotion programs can exert a positive impact on individual health and may also offer an employer such incentives as decreased absenteeism, reduced disability costs, fewer accidents, and greater productivity as well as some long-term potential for containing health care costs. However, hospitals must be cautious in their promises to businesses concerning health promotion's potential for cost containment. A number of variables such as the degree of management's commitment to the program, employee trust or distrust of management's intent, and the quality of health promotion programs and staff can affect the results of health promotion programs. There is also some question as to whether positive results can be sustained over long periods; for example, can a smoking cessation program with a one-year cessation rate of 70 percent maintain that record, or will its success rate drop if more "hard-core" smokers participate in the program? In looking at reported improvements in job performance, some special caution is justified: Is the health promotion program the reason for the improvement, or is it that management has begun to pay attention to employee health?

There is little evidence available on whether health promotion can, in the long run, have much impact on containing the rise in medical care costs. It is difficult to obtain hard data on the cost-effectiveness of health promotion programs in the work place because of the short time that most of these programs have existed. In theory, healthy individuals should have fewer illnesses and thus have lower medical care costs. Whether this happens in fact has yet to be demonstrated for large segments of the population.

Although it may take many years before health promotion programs reduce employers' health care costs, many employers are willing to invest in them because they believe that their greatest value is in improving employees' health and well-being, which in turn will lead to increased productivity. Willis Goldbeck, director of the Washington Business Group on Health, notes that health promotion programs can be viewed as employee benefits that build employee morale and facilitate retention of good workers. "Wellness at the work site," states Goldbeck, "is an expression of a growing awareness among employers that there are ways to address today's health and medical care problems by the direct education and participation of the most important person: each one of us, as individuals, having the opportunity to exercise informed self-responsibility" (ref. 20).

REFERENCES

1. *Roget's International Thesaurus of Quotations.* 1980.

2. American Hospital Association. *The Hospital's Responsibility for Health Promotion.* Chicago: AHA, 1979.

3. U.S. Department of Health, Education and Welfare. *Healthy People: The Surgeon General's Report on Health Promotion and Disease Prevention.* Washington, DC: HEW, 1979, p. 119.

4. O'Hanlon, James. Mirror, mirror, on the wall. *Forbes.* 122:96, Oct. 2, 1978.

5. Whitaker, Joseph D. *Washington Post.* Mar. 1, 1977, p. 1.

6. *Wall Street Journal.* Aug. 11, 1978, p. 18.

7. Berry, Charles A. *Good Health for Employees.* Washington, DC: Health Insurance Institute, 1981.

8. Goldbeck, Willis B., and Kiefhaber, Anne K. Wellness: the new employee benefit. *Voluntary Effort Quarterly.* 2:1-3, Dec. 1980.

9. Sehnert, Keith W., and Tillotson, John K. *How Business Can Promote Good Health for Employees and Their Families.* Washington, DC: National Chamber Foundation, 1978, p. 17.

10. U.S. Department of Health and Human Services. *Smoking Tobacco and Health: A Fact Book.* Washington, DC: U.S. Government Printing Office, 1981, p. 15.

11. Labor letter column. *Wall Street Journal.* 62:1, Mar. 16, 1982.

12. Action on Smoking and Health. *ASH Special Report: The Economics of Employee Smoking.* Washington, DC, undated.

13. Kristein, Marvin. How much can business expect to earn from smoking cessation? In: *Smoking and the Workplace.* New

York City: National Interagency Council on Smoking, Fall 1980, p. 9.

14. U.S. Department of Health and Human Services. *Cardiovascular Primer for the Workplace*. Washington, DC: HHS, p. 24.

15. U.S. Department of Health, Education, and Welfare. *Proceedings of the National Conference on Health Promotion Program in Occupational Settings*. Washington, DC: Government Printing Office, 1979.

16. Health Planning Council. *A Practical Guide for Employee Health Promotion Programs*. Madison, WI: Health Planning Council, Feb. 1979, pp. 7 and 40.

17. Stellman, Jeanne M., and Daum, Susan. *Work Is Dangerous to Your Health*. New York City: Vintage, 1973, p. xiii.

18. Piller, Charles. Staying healthy at work. *Medical Self-Care*. 13:6, Summer 1981.

19. Rowe, Laurens M. Are routine spine films on workers in industry cost- or risk-benefit effective? *Journal of Occupational Medicine*. 24:41-43, Jan. 1982.

20. Goldbeck, Willis. Remarks at AHA conference entitled New Business Opportunities for Hospitals: Health Promotion Services for Local Industry, Orlando, FL, Feb. 23-25, 1981.

Chapter 2

Hospital's Perspective

In 1981, a survey conducted by the American Hospital Association reported that 718 hospitals, or 13.3 percent of all AHA member hospitals, were providing some type of health promotion service to local business and industry on a fee-for-service basis (ref. 1). Of that group, 504 (9.3 percent) were conducting wellness, or life-style, programs for local businesses; 388 (7.2 percent) were providing occupational health services to local businesses; and 313 (5.8 percent) were conducting employee assistance programs for business and industry. Although these statistics show that some hospitals are already providing health promotion programs and services to business and industry, many more are trying to decide whether such services are appropriate for their institutions.

The focus of this book is on helping hospitals decide whether they should approach the development of health promotion services for local business and industry as a *planned comprehensive program that is expected to cover its operational and developmental costs, if not generate surplus revenue.* That is the real issue for a hospital today, and it is one that cannot be approached lightly, because selling health promotion services to local business and industry requires a major commitment of financial and human resources over an extended period. Moreover, it is an issue that a hospital's *leadership* must address. Selling health promotion services to local business and industry is not appropriate for all hospitals, and perhaps not even for a majority.

The decision to commit the hospital to a business-oriented approach to providing health promotion programs generally involves the hospital board, top management, and medical staff leadership. To reach that decision, hospital leaders need to examine several questions in the context of the hospital, its medical staff, its financial resources, and the community it serves, including local business and industry:

- Is community health promotion, with particular emphasis on the health needs of local business and industry, part of the hospital's *mission?* If not, should it be?
- What are the *benefits* for the hospital, the community at large, and local business and industry of participating in health promotion programs?
- Are consumers and local business and industry *ready* for health promotion efforts?

This chapter deals broadly with these questions.

Mission

In 1979 the Surgeon General's report, *Healthy People,* noted that "further improvements in the health of the American people can and will be achieved —not alone through increased medical care and greater health expenditures—but through a renewed national commitment to efforts designed to prevent disease and to promote health" (ref. 2). That same year, the *AHA Environmental Assessment of the Hospital Industry,* which examined changes in society and hospitals for the 1980s, predicted a fundamental expansion of hospitals' missions: "Effective responses [to a changing society] by hospitals will require development of preventive programs, whether through screening, education, or immunization, that will help reduce utilization of inpatient services and reduce the incidence of diseases that are difficult to treat successfully after they have occurred. . . . The role of the health care delivery system will be defined increasingly in terms of prevention and maximizing of the ability of the individual to maintain or improve health. The market for hospital-based health promotion and disease prevention programs for businesses and community groups will continue to expand" (ref. 3).

Some hospitals are responding to the idea of expanding the hospital's mission by revising their mission statements. In its mission statement, a hospital board defines the hospital's reason for being, designates its principal services and primary service area, and sets the parameters for growth and long-range planning. A decade ago, a genuine commitment to health promotion was rare in hospital mission statements. Today, that commitment is becoming more common, because of a growing recognition of the need to expand the hospital's focus beyond the provision of acute medical care.

For example, Porter Memorial Hospital, Denver, Colorado, includes the following institutional goals in its mission statement:

- To promote high-level wellness as the ultimate objective of all hospital-based health and medical services
- To provide health maintenance, preventive care, acute care, and rehabilitation after illness

- To view patients as whole persons, respecting their physical, emotional, social, and spiritual needs
- To provide and maintain special health education services to the patient and the community

Another example is the mission statement of St. Vincent's Hospital in Indianapolis, which revised its mission statement in the late 1970s when the hospital moved from its inner city location to the city's north side, thus altering its patient flow and service area. In its mission statement, the hospital specified its intention "to develop a major thrust in preventive health care programs" (ref. 4). On the basis of this identified mission, the hospital leased 8,900 square feet of store space in a suburban shopping plaza in 1979 and opened a wellness center. A full-time director and receptionist were hired to provide 30 fitness-oriented programs. Total program attendance has been so large that the hospital expects the wellness center to break even within four years. None of this would have happened if the hospital leadership had not first committed the institution to a mission broader than acute inpatient care (ref. 5).

In some cases, a decision to use the hospital's resources to promote health has come about as a result of a commitment by the hospital's governing board or informal assurances of support from key hospital leaders. The Good Health Program at Skokie Valley Community Hospital, Skokie, Illinois, came about from a board-level commitment (ref. 6). In another instance, W. Meade Stockdell Jr., chairman of the board of Lexington County Hospital, West Columbia, South Carolina, is quoted as saying that his institution has a "civic responsibility to keep the citizens of Lexington County well" (ref. 6).

Benefits

The benefits of health promotion can be examined from the perspective of the hospital, the consumer, and local industry. The priorities assigned to potential benefits will differ from community to community and from hospital to hospital.

Benefits for the *hospital* may include the following:

- Improve the health of the hospital's own employees as a result of first developing programs for the hospital's staff before offering them to industry. This is particularly important because hospitals are often hazardous places in which to work. Hospital workers sustain 40 percent more work-related injuries than employees in any other industry (ref. 7). Some of the hazards of hospital work include infections transmitted from patients, puncture wounds from syringes, exposure to toxic chemicals (including pharmaceuticals, anesthetics, disinfectants, solvents, and polishes), chronic exposure to low-level ionizing radiation, and sprains and back injuries from lifting heavy equipment and patients. Back problems account for as many as half of all worker compensation claims filed by hospital workers (ref. 8). Other less apparent but equally hazardous health problems can result from the emotional stress of constantly dealing with life and death situations and decisions. Stress-related health problems among hospital staff can result in physical and emotional burnout, chronic fatigue, depression, and other psychological illnesses.

- Establish the hospital as a center for health in the community.
- Build good relationships with local business and industry and strengthen the hospital's involvement with community business leaders.
- Increase inpatient referrals to the hospital or to physicians for follow-up care as a result of screening programs conducted at the work site.
- Increase non-patient-care revenues, a particularly important concern because third-party reimbursement often covers only a limited range of health education services.
- Provide opportunities for health care professionals to increase their job satisfaction, expand their talents, and apply new techniques for improving health.

Benefits for the *community* may include the following:
- Improve the health of individuals in the community
- Provide a more comprehensive approach to health care
- Provide easier access to preventive services by making programs available at the work site

Benefits for *business* may include the following:
- Improve the health of employees and family members
- Improve employee morale
- Reduce absenteeism
- Reduce long-range expenditures for health care
- Improve productivity
- Provide incentive for recruiting new employees
- Establish community goodwill

Market Readiness

Before a new service can be effectively marketed, the anticipated buyer must be ready for an innovative product. This admonition is particularly important in health promotion, given the slow growth of the preventive medicine movement from the 1940s to the 1970s.

One of the more common arguments against health promotion is that consumers really do not care much about changing their health behavior. Several national surveys give critical insights into this issue (refs. 9 and 10). Individual hospitals also have conducted local surveys to gauge consumer and industry attitudes toward personal health issues as well as toward the hospital as a potential health promotion resource.

The readiness of consumers to accept more self-responsibility for their health was one of the considerations of a 1978-79 study conducted by General Mills. It found that although more Americans were "concerned" rather than "complacent" about their health, only a minority were committed to positive health behavior change (ref. 9).

Another nationwide survey of public attitudes, conducted in 1978 by Louis Harris for Pacific Mutual Life, confirmed the ambivalent findings of the General Mills study (ref. 10). On the one hand, the survey found increased interest and knowledge among Americans regarding personal health concerns. For example, over a five-year span, the number of persons who recognized that it is possible for someone to have high blood pressure without apparent symptoms rose from 30 to 57 percent. The number who knew about the role of excessive salt in hypertension grew from 37 to 61 percent (ref. 10). This increase in knowledge has, in turn, affected the behavior of many individuals. The percentage of the population who have their blood pressure checked every six months or more has increased from 57 percent to 65 percent. The survey also found an increase in the number of individuals actually taking self-responsibility for their own health in other areas as well. The number of Americans involved in regular exercise has increased sharply to 37 percent. And although 57 million Americans still smoke, 20 percent of all adults—some 31 million persons—say they have stopped smoking (ref. 10). On the other hand, the survey also found that for many Americans, "knowledge is not enough." Seven of 10 smokers recognize the risk of lung cancer yet still smoke (ref. 10). Most overweight persons do not follow a weight-reduction diet, and two of every five Americans believe they should exercise more but do not (ref. 10).

The receptivity of employees to health promotion interventions at the work site appears enthusiastic. The Harris survey found that if an employer or the spouse's employer offered a free, preventive health screening program, 43 percent of employees were "very likely" to participate and 21 percent were "somewhat likely." If a $5 per month fee were charged, the responses of those who were "very likely" dropped to 28 percent. Half of the respondents indicated they were likely to participate at the work site in free counseling on nutrition, obesity, stress, and fitness (ref. 10).

According to the Harris survey, business and labor interest was also promising, if not overwhelming. Between 23 and 39 percent of business leaders said they would be likely to adopt a health promotion program for employees, even if it cost $5 per employee per month. Between 26 and 34 percent of union leaders expressed similar support (ref. 10).

Do these statistics indicate enough consumer and business interest to support a hospital's commitment to health promotion at the work site? Are consumers ready? Are local employers ready? Are there sufficient benefits for the hospital, whether those benefits are increased revenues, increased patient referrals, or something else? These are questions that individual hospital leaders must answer as they determine whether to commit resources of their organizations to developing health promotion programs for local business and industry. The following chapters will identify the necessary steps that a hospital should take in order to answer these questions.

REFERENCES

1. American Hospital Association. Special survey on selected hospital topics. Unpublished survey, AHA, Chicago, 1981.
2. Department of Health, Education, and Welfare. *Healthy People: The Surgeon General's Report on Health Promotion and Disease Prevention.* Washington, DC: HEW, 1979, p. 31.
3. American Hospital Association. *AHA Environmental Assessment of the Hospital Industry.* Chicago: AHA, 1980.
4. Maryland Hospital Education Institute, compiler. *Hospital-Sponsored Ambulatory Care: The Governing Board's Role.* Chicago: AHA, 1980, pp. 12-14.
5. *The Ryan Advisory.* Oct. 1980, p. 3.
6. Mabley, Jack. From brownies to carrot sticks; a community health education story. *Trustee.* 32:21-24, Aug. 1979.
7. Stellman, Jeanne M., and Daum, Susan. *Work Is Dangerous to Your Health.* New York City: Vintage, 1973, p. xv.
8. Hospital work: hazardous to your health. *Medical Self-Care.* 13:12-13, Summer 1981.
9. General Mills. *American Family Report, 1978-1979: Family Health in an Era of Stress.* Minneapolis: General Mills, Inc., 1979.
10. Health maintenance survey commissioned by Pacific Mutual Life Insurance Co., and conducted by Louis Harris Associates, Inc. Nov. 1978.

Chapter 3
Employer's Perspective

"Corporate self-interest in growth and profits, coupled with a sense of social and community responsibility, have caused employers to reassess their influence upon health care financing and delivery" (p. 2 of ref. 1). So says the Washington Business Group on Health (WBGH), whose 200 corporate members provide health care benefits to nearly 50 million employees, dependents, and retirees.

Employer involvement in health care was, until recently, relatively indirect. Employers footed the bill for expanding health care benefit packages, provided some in-plant medical and accident prevention services, and served on the boards of hospitals and other health care agencies. Now, an increasing number of employers, both public and private, are taking steps to intervene more directly and overtly in the life-styles of employees and their families and in their decisions about health care. For the most part, this heightened employer involvement is tempered with respect for personal privacy and an emphasis on voluntary decision making by employees. Even these restraints, however, cannot disguise the growing resolve of employers to assume a more aggressive stance with regard to health.

This increased involvement by employers in health is based on a variety of motivations. Although the objectives differ in importance among employers, the primary focus is reduction of medical care costs through decreased utilization of medical services and increased use of alternative delivery models, such as ambulatory surgery and prepaid health care plans. In addition, employers may be motivated by the belief that improved employee health can lead to improved productivity, reduced absenteeism, and reduced disability costs. Some employer health programs came about because of a personal commitment to wellness by a member of top management, whereas other employers are responding to a sense of social responsibility. Finally, some employers develop special health promotion and health care initiatives in order to improve their public image, bolster their employee recruitment efforts, or match a competitor's program. Given this breadth of motivating factors, it is not surprising that recent employer initiatives involving health do not fit neatly into what hospitals might call "health promotion."

The WBGH identifies six of the most common types of employer programs (ref. 1). Their terminology is instructive for hospitals seeking to market to local industry.

- *Improved health awareness.* Employers are disseminating health information through pay envelopes, posters, nutritional signs in the cafeteria, and special events, such as health fairs and lunch-hour health speakers.
- *Life-style modification.* Employers are sponsoring a wide range of wellness and fitness programs, including smoking cessation, weight control, aerobic dancing, and stress management. Some firms have exercise tracks and gymnasiums, and others make special arrangements with nearby recreational facilities.
- *Risk identification.* Employers have long provided or required preemployment and preplacement physicals. Increasingly, they are supporting specific illness screening, health risk appraisals, and screening for toxic substances as required by federal and local laws. High-risk employees are then referred to external resources for appropriate medical counseling or treatment.
- *Enhanced capability to cope with personal problems.* Employee assistance programs provide counseling and referral for employees with problems involving alcoholism, drug abuse, and other personal difficulties.
- *Wise utilization of medical benefits.* Many employers are supporting both voluntary and mandatory surgical second-opinion programs. Others are modifying benefit packages to encourage ambulatory surgery and outpatient care as alternatives to more costly inpatient and emergency treatment.
- *More healthy work environment.* Often under strong regulatory stimulus, employers are establishing stronger safety practices in the work place and are revising hazardous work practices.

Considerations

"Wellness programs are not a fad; they are a growing part of the American landscape," says Willis Goldbeck, director of the WBGH (ref. 2). However, Goldbeck and others add that the increasing business interest in health cannot be translated automatically into sales of hospital-sponsored health promotion programs. Business interest in health has been on the upswing for several years, but hospital chief executive officers have not been swamped with calls for help from local business and industry. Indeed, a 1978 WBGH survey showed that hospitals and doctors were among the last resources to which business and industry look for help in health promotion (ref. 2).

The way in which employers view hospitals and health care issues is critical to planning how to effectively market health promotion services to local business and industry. Many vendors and commercial companies as well as individual entrepreneurs are knocking on the employer's door offering health wares. Hospitals face much competition in the marketplace.

Return on Investment

Some employers considering a health promotion program are likely to place first priority on return on investment. If the company invests in this product or service, what is the payback on the investment? How long will it take to see that return? What can the company anticipate in terms of results? When trying to answer these concerns, the hospital should be cautious about making promises of improved health, lower absenteeism, and improved productivity. Although many questions may be raised about the relationship between health promotion and the reduction of a company's health care expense, many corporate decisions to implement programs are made on an emotional basis. A key executive may have a personal interest in employee health and need little financial data to convince him or her that health promotion services are needed. It is important to know what is paramount to the buyer.

Hospital Credibility

How much confidence will an employer have in a hospital that is developing health promotion services? Part of the answer will depend on that hospital's credibility. Does the hospital provide the program it is selling to its own employees? What are the results? What is the hospital's track record in health promotion? Does the hospital have a strong patient education program? Do the hospital's doctors and nurses encourage the same kind of individual responsibility in their practices that they seek to promote among the employer's work force? Does the hospital medical staff participate in health promotion programs and adhere to healthy life-style practices? In essence, the question is: "Do you practice what you preach?" The hospital seeking to market to local industry must be prepared to answer that question.

Competitive Programs

One employer's attitudes were well expressed by Karl D. Bays, chairman of American Hospital Supply Corporation (AHSC), Evanston, Illinois. From the perspective of a businessman who employs 29,000 persons and is a member of three hospital boards, Bays said: "You don't have to prove to me that it's better to prevent illness and injury than to pay for medical care. Nor do you have to prove to me that individuals who use most of that medical coverage are apt to be the ones who smoke the most, drink the most, or eat the most. I welcome your efforts to promote health. But approval of a concept doesn't guarantee acceptance of a program. There are some things you will have to prove to business people. American Hospital Supply recently approved a $160,000 health promotion program for employees at our corporate headquarters. What sold us on this program was its potential impact on both medical care costs and employee productivity. We're buying the hospitals' programs only when they're competitive, that is, when the hospitals can demonstrate that they have the expertise to be effective and efficient with their health promotion services" (ref. 2).

The American Hospital Supply Corporation has contracted with several local hospitals to implement a health risk factor screening and education program for their Chicago office staff. The company plans to expand the employee health program to other divisions of AHSC around the country by using local community hospitals to conduct screening and education programs.

Next Steps

The market for selling health promotion services to employers exists. Businesses are concerned about the impact of employee life-style on health care costs and have demonstrated a readiness to act. However, economic conditions may limit their readiness to invest and may increase their demands for cost-effectiveness data before purchase. Concepts such as wellness require further definition, and cost-effectiveness measures are sketchy, but the market opportunity is clear.

"One thing that will not change is the need for workers to be healthy," Goldbeck asserts. "Health promotion in that sense is a timeless product. It won't suddenly become good to be obese or stressed. Changes in medical technology won't alter a person's need or desire to be healthy" (ref. 3).

The extent to which hospitals penetrate this market remains to be seen. "Marketing with integrity, not selling, is the only way for a hospital to sell health promotion services to employers," says Goldbeck (ref. 3).

REFERENCES

1. Washington Business Group on Health. *Health Promotion in the Community: A Guide to Working with Employers.* Washington, DC: WBGH, Fall 1980.

2. Bays, Karl D. Remarks at AHA conference entitled New Business Opportunities for Hospitals: Health Promotion Services for Local Industry, Orlando, FL, Feb. 23-25, 1981.
3. Goldbeck, Willis. Remarks at AHA conference entitled New Business Opportunities for Hospitals: Health Promotion Services for Local Industry, Orlando, FL, Feb. 23-25, 1981.

Chapter 4

Market-Oriented Approach to Planning

The process of planning health promotion services for local business and industry differs in a fundamental respect from much of what characterizes planning of other hospital services. Traditionally, hospital planning of inpatient services has been able to count on fairly predictable, slowly changing population trends, such as an aging population in need of hospital care. A hospital can influence its traditional health care market through physician recruitment and ambulatory care programs. Although some hospitals have been economically hurt by territorial invasions of freestanding surgery centers, emergency care centers, and competing hospitals, administrators are seldom surprised by these developments. Hospital chief executive officers do not look out their windows one morning and see an ambulatory surgical center open for business. Market changes generally can be foreseen, and contingency plans can be made.

On the other hand, selling to business and industry is a free-market activity that requires the application of marketing principles. As a vendor in the free marketplace, the hospital will be affected by frequent or rapid shifts in interests, demand, and competition. Competing vendors have no respect for turf. They may also be willing to compete on price. Moreover, services in the marketplace are vulnerable to economic fluctuations. An economic downturn may mean local employers have less money to invest in health care services, which they may see as a fringe benefit that is not crucial to their business.

Marketing is based on the exchange principle: The sale of goods or services is really an exchange between two parties, in which each party gives the other something of value so that a mutually beneficial exchange takes place. The sale of health promotion services to business and industry requires such an exchange. A business expects such values as healthier, more productive workers, lower absenteeism, and perhaps reduced premiums for health insurance, although the long-run impact of health promotion on cost containment still remains to be proved. In return, the hospital expects to help improve the community's state of health and to be paid in cash for doing so.

Until recently, the exchange relationship between a hospital and local business and industry was simple. Employers paid all or part of their employees' insurance premiums. When workers were sick, the doctor sent them to the hospital. Hospital services were a *must* exchange, that is, the local firm had no choice but to buy.

However, when a hospital seeks to offer health promotion services to local firms, a hospital enters a *maybe* exchange. A local company does not have to buy at all, and even if it does, there are many purveyors, such as fitness centers, alcohol treatment programs, and testing services, to choose from in the health promotion marketplace.

Because the purchase of health promotion services concerns a maybe and not a must exchange, the hospital needs to consider the principles of marketing before undertaking the planning and development of such services. In *Marketing Health Care*, MacStravic says that there is a "necessity for the health organization to plan and manage an exchange between itself and other interested parties. The concept of marketing focuses on this exchange and any change in an exchange relationship which is desired by the organization, needed by the community, or both. Whenever a health organization finds itself in a position where it wishes to alter an exchange relationship with physicians, patients, supporters, employees, regulatory agencies, etc., the concepts of marketing may be used to its benefit" (ref. 37).

The planning process described in this chapter is a market-oriented, or client-centered, approach whereas most hospital planning results from a service-centered approach. The distinction is subtle but critical. Service-centered planning assumes that if there is a medical need, then consumers will use the service. In client-centered planning, needs do not necessarily or automatically result in the purchase of services. The client's decision to purchase services is based on a series of decisions. Client-centered planning recognizes that a buyer must:

- See the need for a given service. For example, employers must recognize that there are alcoholic employees in their work force.
- Decide that the need is important enough to address. For example, are alcoholic workers causing decreased productivity or placing an undue burden on supervisors?
- Agree that the work place is an appropriate site for handling the problem.
- Understand how the hospital's services will help meet this need.

- Decide whether to choose the hospital's services over those of other competitors.

It is also important to note that the hospital must now focus on a new client, business and industry, rather than on physicians, other health care professionals, or patients, the groups that the hospital has traditionally perceived as the primary purchaser of services. By broadening their client market to include business and industry, hospitals are subject to the same risks as any other entrepreneur.

Planning Process

To compete in a free market, the hospital must plan carefully to determine whether it should be offering health promotion services to business and industry. The planning process suggested here includes seven steps divided into a *research and analysis phase* and an *action planning phase:*

Research and Analysis Phase
1. General assessment
2. Marketing orientation
3. Business and industry assessment
4. Hospital assessment

Action Planning Phase
5. Building a program
6. Planning for sales

These steps represent an organized planning framework that individual hospitals will need to adjust for their specific situations. It is not intended to show hospitals how to implement a specific health promotion program. Rather, it provides a process to help the hospitals make decisions about whether to provide health promotion services to business and industry.

Step 1. General Assessment

The general assessment is a critical step often overlooked in a planning process. The general assessment step is designed to determine:
- Whether it is appropriate for the hospital to consider providing health promotion services to business and industry
- Whether there are potential clients to support health promotion services
- What kinds of health promotion activities have been offered successfully by other providers.

This general assessment step is important because it can help ensure that the hospital does not make mistaken assumptions about the hospital's internal and external environment. During the general assessment, the hospital must consider its mission and leadership, the benefits it will gain from health promotion programs, the readiness of labor and industry to accept such programs, and the existing and proposed programs of possible competitors.

Mission and Leadership

The hospital should examine its mission statement and long-range plan to see what they say about health promotion, community outreach, and serving local business and industry. Developing health promotion services for industry does not fit into the mission and long-range plan of every hospital. The idea of providing health promotion services to business and industry should be discussed with board members, top administration, and medical staff leaders to ascertain if they accept the argument, advanced by the Surgeon General of the United States and by AHA, that hospitals must expand from an acute care mission to a broader focus of promoting health (refs. 1 and 2). If the leaders in the hospital do not accept this view, then some education will be needed to enhance their awareness and understanding of these issues. The hospital must determine if it can afford the business risk of providing a new type of service and if it has the resources to commit to the development of new products. In short, the leadership of the hospital must determine early in the process whether it is ready to become seriously involved in marketing health promotion services to business and industry.

Benefits

One way to determine the hospital's readiness is to determine what the hospital wishes to gain from health promotion services. Many of the reasons for becoming involved in health promotion were mentioned in chapter 2. As part of the planning process, those reasons should be applied to the specific institution. The hospital should review its long-range planning documents and the services it already has under way to ascertain whether a health promotion program would complement other efforts or compete for resources.

Health promotion programs can make an important contribution to containing individual, community, and, in the long run, institutional health care costs. Health promotion programs are designed to encourage individuals to take greater responsibility for their own health and, by preventing disease and improving their well-being, to reduce individual health care costs. Health promotion programs also can be an effective means to improve the image of the hospital, and if carefully planned and developed, they have the potential to generate revenue and to develop new markets.

Any new service of the hospital has the potential to influence the use of existing health care resources. Health promotion programs can be designed to increase referrals to physicians affiliated with the hospital; decrease or increase the use of hospital services, such as emergency departments, ambulatory centers, or day surgeries; and increase the use of the hospital for inpatient services. Because health promotion programs seek to inform, educate, and encourage involvement in health care decisions, the participants may be positively influenced to choose the hospital when care is needed. Possibly the most compelling reason for hospitals to consider making a greater commitment to health promotion is that the institution has a major responsibility to the health of the entire community. Some hospitals believe that their involvement in health promotion for their own employees, a logical starting place for new programs, not only improves the health of the work force, but also provides a recruitment benefit. As part of the planning process, it is important to recognize these health and nonhealth benefits and to set priorities for them.

Industry and Labor Readiness

The hospital must determine whether local employers and unions are ready to become engaged in health promotion services at the work site. To make this determination, the hospital should get answers to the following questions about employers' and unions' existing involvement in health: Do any of their leaders or members serve on hospital or other health care agency boards? Have they made statements about health care costs or health promotion? Do they have corporate goals or objectives regarding employee health? Do they support community health organizations, such as the American Cancer Society? Have any employers begun work-site health promotion activities? Is the local economy healthy enough to permit investment in health promotion? What are the major health problems (for example, alcoholism, smoking) present in the working population? Do employers and unions seem to be aware of these problems, or is some education required to build their awareness and understanding?

Programs of Others

What can be learned from the experiences of others? At this point it may not be clear what programs the hospital should consider. The hospital decision maker responsible for this assessment process should review chapter 1 to see whether the effective programs described there are feasible for the hospital. A computerized literature search, such as the Health Planning and Administration Data Base that is available through the Library of the American Hospital Association, Asa S. Bacon Memorial, or NTIS (National Technical Information Service), where federal contractors file project reports, can provide valuable information on the effectiveness, implementation strategies, and evaluation techniques reported by health promotion programs at the work site.

Other more informal ways of obtaining information on effective work-site programs are to:

- Check the local public library for reports in the popular literature, such as newspapers and business magazines.
- Call the local chamber of commerce to see if it knows of local business and industry involvement in health promotion.
- Write or call hospitals in other areas who already have begun these activities. AHA's Center for Health Promotion can provide some examples.
- Talk with key staff and board members at the hospital. Many may have heard their colleagues refer to activities that are being conducted elsewhere.

An inventory of effective program ideas should be developed. These references will be helpful if the hospital chooses to proceed with the planning process.

Key Questions

To determine whether the hospital should continue with the planning process, a key hospital decision maker should answer a number of questions. If the answer to each question is yes, then the hospital should proceed to the next planning step. If the answer to any question is no, the hospital decision maker needs to investigate further or take action to change the answer to yes before proceeding with the planning process. The questions are:

- Is health promotion for business and industry an appropriate service for the hospital? Yes _____ No _____
- Have the leaders of the hospital shown any interest in a health promotion project for business and industry?
  Yes _____ No _____
- Does the hospital's mission statement embrace health promotion concepts? Yes _____ No _____
- Does this project complement other long-range plans of the hospital?
  Yes _____ No _____
- Are the payoffs substantial? Yes _____ No _____
- Has local business and industry shown an interest in health affairs?
  Yes _____ No _____

Step 2. Marketing Orientation

This step helps hospital leaders ensure that their thinking is actually market oriented and not focused on hospital-perceived needs. Looking at a health promotion service from the perspective of the employer can give the hospital a different outlook on marketing than it had when planning other new hospital programs. The ability to operate from the client's perspective is crucial in developing services that will meet the needs of clients and provide the hospital with the benefits it seeks.

Client's Perception

Most employers have little or no experience with employee assistance programs; wellness, or life-style, programs; or health-promotion-oriented occupational health services. As a result, the employer will see the hospital's services as a new product or an innovation. Professional marketers have identified a number of elements in what a client perceives as an innovation. As a consultant to hospitals in the field of health promotion, Robert Rotanz, president, Rotanz Associates, Berkeley, New Jersey, identifies five elements that are particularly critical in marketing health promotion services (ref. 4):

- *Benefit.* How will the client perceive the benefit or advantage to his or her company? What education might be necessary to have the client accept the hospital's perception of the benefit?
- *Compatibility.* Is the service or product compatible with the values, method of operation, and purpose of the client?
- *Complexity.* Will the client have difficulty either in understanding the product or service or implementing it within his or her organization? Will the complexity of the program or service outweigh the benefit?
- *Testability.* Can the client test the program or service before making a major commitment to its use?
- *Observability.* Can the client see the results of the program in a setting similar to his or her own?

The following examples illustrate how these concepts can be applied to health promotion services:

- *What's the benefit?* Employers see benefits in terms of return on investment. Will an investment in a health promotion service reduce other expenditures? For example, will an employee assistance program result in reduced absenteeism, improved morale, greater productivity, and lower utilization of medical services? Will exercise and fitness programs make employees more vigorous and productive?
- *Will it fit in?* Any product or service must be compatible with the client's business. A smoking cessation course is probably not salable to a tobacco producer, and classes on proper lifting techniques may not be appropriate for clerical or sales personnel.
- *Can it be understood easily?* A health promotion service should not be too complex. A person who buys a car wants to know how to drive it, not how it works. Similarly, an employer does not want to know the theory behind a weight control course, but rather how many employees will enroll in the course, whether it will take time away from work, and what results can be expected.
- *Can it be tested?* Employers may ask if a new service can be tried or demonstrated. They may want to know if they have to buy a whole package of services or if they can purchase separate program com-

ponents? For example, must they buy an entire health screening and education program, or can they purchase only the weight control and stress management segments? They may also be interested in offering a program to only one group within the organization, such as top management and then later provide the program to hourly employees.

- *Who has done it? What were the results?* The hospital needs to determine how it can test potential health promotion services in order to develop product credibility and allow potential clients to observe the program as it is being implemented. This is where a hospital's program for its own staff is critical. For example, if a hospital has an employee assistance program for its own employees, it can provide data on how many employees with problems were identified, referred to counseling or treatment, and actually counseled or entered treatment and what the outcome was in terms of their present employment status. The hospital may also have data on the effects of the program on absenteeism and performance. If the health promotion service the employer wants is not appropriate for the hospital's employees, the hospital may need to offer a sample pilot program to demonstrate its effectiveness to the potential client. Some activities, such as a screening program, can often be viewed at a local community health fair. Educational and exercise classes can be conducted on a sample basis to allow a potential client to observe and evaluate their effectiveness.

Using the five elements of benefit, compatibility, complexity, testability, and observability as a framework for proceeding, the hospital should identify staff members who have the skills needed to plan client-centered activities. Many hospitals may find that they do not have health care professionals on their staff who have been trained in marketing or organizational analysis, and both perspectives will be needed to continue the planning process. If these skills do not exist within the hospital, it may be necessary to look for specialists outside the institution. Once the marketing elements are understood, capable staff have been identified to continue the planning process, and reasonable accommodations for demonstrating the service are made, then the next step is to learn more about potential customers.

Key Questions

To determine whether the hospital should continue with the planning process, a key hospital decision maker should answer a number of questions. If the answer to each question is yes, then the hospital should proceed to the next planning step. If the answer to any question is no, the hospital decision maker needs to investigate further or take action to change the answer to yes before proceeding with the planning process. The questions are:

- Has the hospital examined all elements of the program or service from

the client's perspective? Yes _____ No _____
- Does the hospital have staff or consultants who are knowledgeable about marketing? Yes _____ No _____
- Does the hospital have opportunities to test its health promotion ideas before selling them to others? Yes _____ No _____

Step 3. Business and Industry Assessment

Before a hospital can begin to plan a program, it must identify its potential clients and determine their needs. The hospital needs to determine how many businesses are accessible to the hospital, whether they have common or diverse characteristics and needs, and what services they are most likely to use.

Process for Assessment

The following steps are designed to help identify and contact businesses to determine their specific needs and interests in the hospital's programs. This series of activities outlines a process that can be altered or refined as necessary.

- The hospital should make a tentative decision about the geographic area it chooses to serve. This can be revised if necessary, after more information about local business and industry is available. The hospital may decide to focus on an already well-established service area. In other cases, the local transportation system may influence the service area boundaries. For example, the distance that staff can reasonably be expected to travel in bad weather to provide a program may determine the geographic boundaries.
- After the service area has been determined, a list of the companies in that area should be compiled. Government agencies, local chambers of commerce, and manufacturers' indexes can provide information to help make up this list. Many of these will categorize the companies by size and type of business so that the hospital can chart the range of industries and group the businesses by number of employees.
- The hospital should identify a group of local businesses it would like to contact. In some cases, local branches of larger firms might be eliminated from this list if it is found that decisions about health promotion programs are controlled by the corporate offices. Businesses with fewer than 100 employees might also be eliminated unless a majority of the businesses in the service area are that size and the hospital determines that it wants to offer services to a consortium of small businesses.
- In order to ascertain the potential salability of a new product or service, companies on the list should be surveyed to learn about their perceptions of a new product or service before it is developed. One approach

is to write to all the identified businesses to inform them that a representative from the hospital would like to discuss what their health promotion needs are as well as what potential services the hospital could provide to meet those needs. The letter can be followed by a telephone interview that asks some of the questions described in the interview process later in this step.

- The final step in the business and industry assessment is to conduct a series of structured interviews with carefully selected business representatives. A small group of businesses that will be contacted in person should be selected from the list developed by the hospital. These businesses may be chosen because the hospital has established good relationships with them in the past or because they were particularly responsive and helpful in the telephone interviews. These personal interviews can also be supplemented with less formal group information-gathering sessions. For example, Union Hospital of Lynn, Massachusetts, gave a luncheon for 30 corporate officials to hear their informal views about the current health needs and problems of their employees.

Personal Interviews

At this point, the hospital representative is armed with some preliminary data and background information about business and industry in the area. Now the representative becomes a market researcher. To make the market research effective, he or she should thoroughly plan how to approach an executive or manager in the business or industry to discuss the hospital's health promotion services. The purpose of this interview is to get sound opinions and value judgments from the business manager. Remember that the objective of the personal interview is to gather information, not to disseminate it. The industry manager should not be led to certain conclusions simply because those conclusions fit the hospital's capabilities. Misreadings at this point can lead to future business disappointments and failures.

Robert Rotanz recommends that interviewers plan their entire interaction with the industry manager by asking these questions (ref. 4):

- *Why am I asking?*

    The interviewer must clearly convey the purpose of the interview to the interviewee. For example, the interviewer might say, "Our hospital is seriously considering offering health promotion services to local industry. These services would be available at the work site. As part of our planning process, we're talking to business managers to get a better idea of what you're doing with regard to employee health and what you need. I'm not here today to sell anything, although I may be back in a few months with a specific program to offer you."

- *What do I ask?*

  This section of the interview should initially focus on broad questions about health promotion categories and then proceed to specific areas of interest to the business. The objective of this part of the interview is to encourage responses to the hospital's areas of interest while simultaneously focusing on the client's specific needs.

  It this point, the hospital may have some tentative services in mind. It may already be thinking about offering occupational screening services, for example. However, the interviewer needs to ask some leading questions to test the waters for employee assistance and wellness, or life-style, programs as well. For example, the interviewer might ask the following: "Do you require examinations for new employees or for executives only? Where are physicals done and by whom? What are the costs of your present programs? What happens when a worker is injured on the job? How is treatment handled? What kinds of on-the-job injuries are most common: hearing loss, eye injuries, fractures, or others? Do you have much of a problem with alcoholic employees or drug abusers? How do you deal with these problems? What is the role of supervisors in identifying employees who have personal problems that are affecting their job performance? Do they receive any training in dealing with alcoholism or substance abuse? Do you know what illnesses account for most of the claims for health care benefits by employees (listen especially for illnesses that are linked to health habits)? Do you at present offer any health education information programs aimed at avoiding these problems?"

  The interviewer should describe some health promotion services briefly and try to get a response as to whether the business might be interested in purchasing them. For example, the interviewer might say, "If you were offered a program to help identify, counsel, and refer for treatment employees with personal problems such as alcoholism and drug abuse, would you buy it? How much per employee would you be willing to pay? Would you buy a program to screen your employees for disease and refer those with health risks either to treatment or to health education classes?"

  The interviewer can learn how the company works by asking questions such as the following: "Who makes the decisions here about employee benefits, in-plant medical services, and safety and accident prevention? Whom do we have to sell?" You may have to ask the last question specifically for each type of program the hospital is considering developing. For example, the medical director might purchase an occupational health program, but the chief executive officer may make the decision about an employee assistance program.

The interviewer can learn about the company's attitudes toward the hospital by asking such questions as: "What do you know about us? What do you hear about the care given to your employees and dependents in our hospital and clinics?"

- *How do I ask?*

A totally unstructured interview may be cozy and relaxed, but it is rarely informative and often leaves interviewees unsatisfied and feeling that their time has been wasted. On the other hand, a highly structured interview may prevent the interviewer from picking up on nuances or unspoken attitudes. The ideal approach is somewhere in between. It enables the interviewer to use the best aspects of both structured and unstructured interviews. The correct approach should be a consistently refined, qualitative approach that touches on each area of health promotion.

It is equally important that the interviewer adjust interviews to account for responses from other meetings. That is, at the completion of each individual interview, the interviewer should be prepared to redesign the questions for any succeeding interviews. It may also be necessary to restructure and redefine questions in terms of the client's needs. Additional interviews will further refine the pattern and begin to build knowledge about which companies will be most receptive to the final products. By conducting 6 to 12 such interviews, the interviewer should be able to discern an emerging pattern of responses that will allow him or her to assess the needs of local business and industry for health promotion or disease prevention programs and services that the hospital could successfully develop and market.

- *Whom do I ask?*

The selection of the level of management and the departments to be approached is significant to the interview process. The interviewer must be sensitive to the personal interests of various managers. Rotanz says, "The chairman of the board may be positive because he is people oriented, the president may be negative because he is responsible for shrinking profits, the personnel manager may be sensitive to increased cost of benefits, and the ultimate manager responsible for the implementation of the program may feel threatened" (ref. 4). Knowledge of the specific company and of organizational behavior is helpful here. The interviewer should anticipate what biases may be built into the responses because of the interviewee's job function or status.

Michael J. Gallagher, vice-president for operations, Swedish American Hospital, Rockford, Illinois, emphasizes the need to interview industry managers in person, not via a mailed questionnaire (ref. 5). His hospital interviewed managers from companies that sent injured or ill employees to the hospital's emergency department and clinics. It also picked companies that had an executive on the hospital's board. The hospital's market research also included discussions with local physicians who received most of the referrals for plant injuries and workers' compensation.

Gallagher urges that market research include interviews not only with top management, but also with the company health nurse and physician, safety director, personnel director, and insurance representative. These individuals may be directly involved with the ultimate program, and their support may be critical in a corporate decision to buy.

- *What do you hear?*

In interviewing employers, there is a danger that interviewees will respond with statements that they think the interviewer wants to hear. Therefore, the interviewer must phrase questions carefully. For example, such questions as "would you buy. . ." demand no commitment. Questions like "will you buy this product from me?" eliminate generalities and demand a yes or no decision from the interviewee. This is one of the difficulties in market research. Inviting and receiving positive comments about a future product or service is different from making the sale.

This difficulty is compounded when the situation is new, unusual, or unique. Such a situation exists when a hospital manager is recommending to a business manager that the hospital design, develop, and market a health promotion service for that business. The business manager may respond positively to health promotion programs in a conversation with a hospital representative, but there may be other considerations and reservations on the part of the business that do not come up in the conversation. These considerations might include lack of conviction, commitment to other projects, skepticism that a hospital can deal with the internal problems of the business or industry, requirements that all projects are internally developed and managed by the business, or concern about the continued financial health of the corporation.

Gallagher says he learned much from his interviews that helped the hospital tailor its occupational health service to the needs of local business and industry (see case study 4 in chapter 6). Many of the industry managers he interviewed put a high priority on physician knowledge, competence, and interest: "Will your doctors come to the plant? We haven't seen some physicians to whom we refer for 10 years." Gallagher found that the companies his hospital contacted wanted timely reports for insurance and workers' compensation purposes. Some wanted work-site environmental assessments to determine occupational hazards, whereas others voiced the need for care of the whole person, not just treatment of on-the-job injuries. Says Gallagher, "Once you hear the responses, you must establish priorities. You can't meet all the needs. Match the business's greatest needs with the hospital's resources" (ref. 3).

Key Questions

To determine whether the hospital should continue with the planning process, a key hospital decision maker should answer a number of questions. If the answer to each question is yes, then the hospital should proceed to the next planning step. If the answer to any question is no, the hospital decision maker needs to investigate further or take action to change the answer to yes before proceeding with the planning process. These questions are:

- Does the hospital's chosen service area include a sizable number of businesses? Yes _____   No _____
- Are there a significant number of businesses that appear to have an interest in employee health issues? Yes _____   No _____
- Are the health concerns and needs of local businesses amenable to health promotion programs? Yes _____   No _____
- Is there any consistency in the needs of businesses in the hospital's chosen service area? Yes _____   No _____

Step 4. Hospital Assessment

Any organization that is planning to expand operations beyond its normal activities must assess the internal impact of such changes. A hospital is an extremely complex organization with a great many resources at its command. It must take a long penetrating look at itself before it moves beyond its traditional mission.

When looking at the opportunities in health promotion, the hospital decision maker must be aware of the attitudes of staff and physicians concerning the hospital's role in health promotion and in providing services to business and industry. Staff and physicians may have misgivings and may voice concerns, such as the following: The hospital is performing its traditional role well so why change; similar programs have been tried before and failed; these programs have been previously offered free as a community service; the hospital is going to look too much like a commercial organization; and competing hospitals offer similar programs.

Although there is no easy answer to the question of how to gain support from physicians and staff, it is best to start by making available ample information about the hospital's goals. Frequent communication, in writing and in person, should help ensure that the motives behind the hospital's providing health promotion services to business and industry are understood, even if not fully accepted. Experience has shown that many of the concerns disappear and the attitudes change once staff and physicians see the quality of the proposed services and their acceptance by business and industry.

In addition to explaining the new role of the hospital, the hospital decision maker must be aware that certain jealousies may occur as a result of the redirection of attention and energy. If other services in the hospital have had the spotlight for several years and that spotlight is now shifted to health promotion, it is natural that the reduced attention to these other services may result in new tensions. Shifting resource allocations in a system in which the competition for new resources is already fierce can add to negative attitudes toward health promotion unless every opportunity is taken to demonstrate how the shift is related to hospital goals.

Hospital Programs and Services

It is vital that the key hospital decision maker objectively assess the capabilities of the services, programs, and facilities within the institution. This assessment must be done without regard to personal loyalties, past involvement in programs, or assumptions about effectiveness that are based on reports from participants or providers. Programs that have been effective as free community services must be carefully reevaluated to determine whether they are appropriate to be offered as purchased services. It is likely that modifications will be required before such programs are salable to business and industry.

One way to begin an analysis of the resources of the hospital is to build a list of all the services related to health promotion that the hospital is already offering, with particular emphasis on programs that are provided as community services or are delivered outside the hospital building. All health promotion services offered to anyone, whether to inpatients, schools, the community, or business, and all ambulatory or outreach programs and inpatient services that may be related to health promotion should be listed. Does the hospital have clinics, neighborhood health care centers, or other ambulatory care programs? These programs may have space or personnel that could be valuable in delivering health promotion services to industry. Does the hospital have patient education as a priority? If so, the resource materials and staff may be key components in building new programs. What programs, such as health fairs, newsletters, speakers' bureaus, and so forth, are offered as community relations services? The contacts from these programs may help the hospital build a client list.

Next it is important to identify the specific resources that are available for the programs listed. Existing resources are not useful if they are overloaded. Building on current programs is not helpful if the services are of poor quality or have not been received well in the community. Be sure the list includes:

- Clinical and educational staff who teach patients and community members

- Staff for diagnostic testing and screening
- Public relations staff to assist with the development and marketing of promotional brochures
- Information sources for health care data or marketing contacts
- Physicians who might serve in planning or advisory capacities
- Clerical staff to assist in scheduling, data collection, and record-keeping functions
- Physical resources, such as space, audiovisual media, and diagnostic equipment
- Health education materials, both print and audiovisuals

At this point, the effectiveness of the programs must be evaluated, and services should be listed in terms of their potential contribution to health promotion activities. Are the services compatible with the hospital's new goals? Are the issues of territoriality so great that cooperative arrangements would not be possible? Is the reputation of the service or program good? What are the problems that would have to be overcome in order to convert the present programs to services for business and industry? Are the services mobile? Will offering a service to business overtax the support services of the hospital? For example, if screening for a specific disease is a component of a health promotion service, would the screening overload the x-ray or laboratory facilities? Much of this evaluation is subjective, but it is crucial that the hospital decision maker know what potential resources are usable.

Programs of Others

What is the competition, past and present, from other hospitals, community health care agencies, and others? Do they have any competitive advantages or disadvantages? It is important to find out what health promotion services are being offered by other hospitals, health maintenance organizations, community clinics, local voluntary health agencies, and public health departments. These local health care providers have information on their programs and any resources that they might have available. Some agencies provide instructors, equipment, and materials on subjects related to their missions. What are the community agencies, such as the YMCA, YWCA, community centers or recreation centers, or local schools, doing about health? Commercial enterprises, such as weight control programs, should also be evaluated. The advertisements in local newspapers should provide some information on what the competition is doing.

At some point in the planning process, a decision about whether the hospital should be in direct competition with other providers or should develop only those programs that are not being offered by others will have to be made. At this stage, however, it is more important to have a complete inventory of programs in direct competition with the one the hospital is planning.

Obstacles and Support

Internal obstacles may be real or perceived and may include resistance by one or more members of top management; lack of staff, space, or capitalization funds; and physician resistance. It is important to pin down the specific reasons for opposition by key staff members. For example, if there is resistance by physicians, is it because of their belief that the services may intrude on their practices, general skepticism about health promotion as a concept, hesitance about hospital involvement at work sites, concern about the ability to control the quality of programs that are offered outside the hospital, or personal disillusionment as a result of their own unsuccessful attempts to change the behavior of patients?

Once the obstacles have been identified, they must be dealt with directly. In addition to having supporters discuss the benefits of health promotion activities, there are several other strategies that can be used to build support:

- A draft statement of health promotion and hospital involvement at the work site can be developed. The statement can be approved by the hospital governing board and used as a focal point for discussions with hospital and medical staffs.
- Those who support the idea of health promotion services can be asked to talk with those who resist it. A physician who is particularly knowledgeable about work-site programs can talk with colleagues who think that providing programs to business and industry is inappropriate for hospitals. One or two staff members who are skeptical about the program can be asked to actively participate on an advisory committee.
- The hospital should find out what benefits from a program would *sell* the opposition and seek their advice on how to build those benefits into the program.
- Everyone who might be affected by the introduction of a program should be kept informed of the planning process as it progresses.

As much attention should be given to the persons who support health promotion as to those perceived as obstacles. A list of key physicians and managers who are ready to help should be developed, and their particular areas of interest should be identified. Those hospital programs that are now successful but were once believed to be marginal ventures should be examined. They can be used as reminders that new programs can pay off. Furthermore, the staff associated with such programs may be the best supporters of new business ventures.

Key Questions

To determine whether the hospital should continue with the planning process, a key hospital decision maker should answer a number of questions. If the answer to each question is yes, then the hospital should proceed to the next planning step. If the answer to any question is no, the hospital decision maker needs to investigate further or take action to change the answer to yes before proceeding with the planning process. These questions are:

- Can the hospital identify how services and programs it offers have contributed to the community? Yes _____ No _____
- Has the hospital developed a list of available resources that might be used in developing a health promotion service or program? Yes _____ No _____
- Has the hospital identified specific obstacles to program development? Yes _____ No _____
- Does the hospital have a plan to overcome the obstacles to its health promotion program? Yes _____ No _____
- Does the hospital have a list of competing services offered in the community? Yes _____ No _____
- Do local business and industry have health promotion needs that are not being served by the competition? Yes _____ No _____

Step 5. Program Building

The research and analysis phase of the planning process has identified why the hospital wishes to pursue a new business venture, focused on the health concerns and needs of local business and industry, and yielded a list of hospital programs and resources that can be useful in the action planning phase. This action planning phase, which consists of this step and step 6 (see page 51), provides guidance on how to build a program to meet the needs of the hospital and local employers.

Selection

If a hospital is to offer services to business and industry, it should start with a program that has the highest potential for success. Therefore, it should look at the health promotion needs most often mentioned during the personal interviews and match them with the most prominent and effective services and resources that are extant in the hospital.

To do this, the hospital should begin by choosing one program that appears to meet client needs and then checking with the goals the hospital has established for entering the health promotion arena. Will the chosen program yield results that are compatible with the hospital's mission and objectives? If not, the hospital must look for another match between the needs of business and industry and potential services provided by the hospital and keep on looking until a program that suits the hospital's goals, the resources available, and the needs of local business and industry is found.

Target Market

The interviews that were conducted with businesses (in step 3) should give the hospital direction in establishing a target for its marketing efforts. Does the planned service appeal to large organizations, or is it a program that is more effective for employers with less than 500 employees? Is the program suited to manufacturing organizations with assembly-line operations that limit the time workers can be away from the line? Would sales efforts be more fruitful if the program were set up for scientific and professional workers only? How many businesses in the selected area are of sufficient size and nature to need the hospital's product?

These questions may seem unimportant at this point, but as soon as the hospital begins to develop the program elements and determine the cost of operations, the wisdom of calculating the size and nature of potential users early in the process will become apparent. For example, if a large number of small employers are being served, delivery costs and the difficulties of offering the program at each work site may put the price of the program beyond the means of employers. Manufacturing firms may be unwilling to pull workers off the line to attend programs that require participants to spend extensive time off the job. Therefore, the design of the program has to be related to the kinds of business and industry in the local area.

Design and Description

The next step is to design and describe the potential program elements as completely as possible. In doing so, the hospital should provide a description of the benefits the company will receive by implementing the program rather than only describing the services it will get. For example, a smoking cessation class is a service; the reduction of smoking-related illness is a benefit.

In designing and describing the elements of the program, it is important to look to the work of others and to the comments made by the businesses and industries that have been interviewed in order to accommodate the wishes of future clients. The following points should be considered when describing the program components:

- Is program implementation designed to be compatible with the needs of the business or industry? For example, can programs be conducted at the work site? Can classes be scheduled before or after working hours?
- Are elements of the program educational? Is it designed for large-group or small-group participation?
- What reports, measurements, or evaluation data will be provided as part of the service? How will the quality of the service be monitored?
- If a local businesses or industry has a medical director, has the hospital considered how that person will be involved in the program, and is this decision acceptable to the prospective client? If not, is

the hospital willing to compromise in order to make a sale?

- Has the hospital determined which elements of the program are integral to its value and cannot be compromised? For example, maintaining the confidentiality of individual employees who have sought help through an employee assistance program is a component that should not be compromised.
- What are the responsibilities of the client? Must the client supply any clerical staff, space, equipment? Has the hospital thought through the advantages and disadvantages of giving some of the control as well as the responsibility for the success or failure of the program to someone within the client organization? How will a coordinator at the work site, who will probably be an employee of the business, interface with the hospital program staff coordinator?

Everything the hospital plans to do should be written down as clearly as possible. Although the preliminary decisions that are made at this point may be modified as implementation begins, it is important to critically examine the viability of the proposed program from the viewpoint of the client. All information about the program should be described and presented in terms of the client's interests and perspective.

Included in the program description should be a list of the resources needed to fully develop, sell, and implement the program. What staff and services will be needed to develop the sales materials? What space, equipment, materials, and staff will be necessary to deliver the program elements to the work site? Who will continue to serve the client, that is, provide reports, give evaluation or measurement data, answer questions, and so forth? These three major issues—development, delivery, and sales and marketing—must be examined throughout the planning process.

Costs

A problem in new business development is that the market for the program is often overestimated and the investments needed to reach the marketplace are usually underestimated. Another common mistake is to assume that existing personnel from one area can be borrowed on a part-time basis and applied to a new business venture without a loss of performance in either area. Probably the greatest mistake in new business development is underestimating time. Because of enthusiasm and a desire to present a positive view to management, the planner frequently minimizes the cost of starting a business. This folly can quickly kill a budding program.

The planner must begin by determining developmental costs. The first thing to do is to estimate the number of days of work needed to fully develop the program or service. Then the salaries of the individuals who will be providing these services must be calculated. If the hospital decides to use outside contractors to provide these services, it must get an estimate of the costs from them. The hospital may want to include in its calculation of costs the space and utilities that the staff is using during this planning phase. All direct costs that can be identified with the developmental phase of the planning process should be included.

If a new program with which local business and industry are not familiar is being developed, the hospital can probably assume several months of sales activities before making its first sale. If it is developing a service that business and industry know and use, that time may be reduced.

The costs of the sales force and the supporting sales materials that it will require must also be calculated. Is the hospital going to develop a brochure that describes its service? Will this brochure be mailed to local industries? What will the postal charges for this mailing be? Will the hospital advertise in the media? What about the out-of-pocket expenses for local travel for the hospital staff responsible for program sales?

Next, the costs of the actual delivery of the product must be calculated. Direct costs such as salaries, supplies, and equipment must be included, plus whatever chargebacks the hospital wishes to use to cover administrative costs and space and utility allocations.

Working with the hospital accountants at this point is important because the price of the service will be established on the basis of these estimated costs. If any costs are omitted, the price that will be established will not be correct, and it is awkward to adjust the price once a new service has been introduced.

Pricing

The price of a product should be based on the best available cost estimates and should include marketing, program development, implementation, and profit. In addition to being competitive with similar services, the price of the product is related to the delivery format and the needs of the hospital. For example, a program that is offered on a one-time basis to an employer and is not sensitive to the number of participants could be priced at a flat sum to be paid when the program is delivered. A service such as health screening, examinations, or risk appraisals might have a price per participant plus a management fee paid in advance to cover the necessary charges for setting up the program. Ongoing programs may have a combination of these pricing schemes, or they may have quarterly charges or fees per hour of service.

At this point in the planning process, the hospital may not be able to establish a firm price for its program because some of the costs are still unknown. However, it is a good idea to set a price range that can be used when testing the program on the market.

Planning Example

An example illustrating how to design a program following the suggestions outlined in step 5 might prove helpful. Memorial Hospital (a hypothetical institution) is interested in providing health promotion programs to business and industry. The hospital would like to increase the use of its present services and provide its physicians with a continuing supply of patients. The staff of Memorial conducted a survey of local business and industry and found that there were three major concerns:

- Inpatient costs were soaring and the employers wanted to find a way to reduce the number of hospital admissions by their employees.
- Absenteeism seemed quite high, and the patterns of absence indicated possible alcohol, drug, and stress problems in the employee population.
- Some industries were concerned about the effects of toxic materials on the workers.

After analyzing the hospital's strengths and matching them against the needs of business, Memorial Hospital staff found that the first concern of local business and industry, to reduce hospital admissions, is not one the hospital is prepared to handle. Monitoring inpatient costs and length of stay is a project already under way because of hospital management concerns. Memorial knows that it cannot respond to the third concern identified by the survey because it has no services, programs, or resources related to toxicology, and although such a service could be developed, there appear to be too few industries that are genuinely interested. Fortunately, Memorial operates an inpatient alcoholism treatment center, provides outpatient counseling in alcohol and drug abuse, and has a fine psychiatric service. The treatment facility and the alcohol and drug abuse service are capable of handling more clients. Therefore, it seems logical that the first program Memorial should develop is an employee assistance program.

Reviewing the notes made during the industry assessment, staff members find that the greatest interest in this service is from small businesses. An employee assistance program that would be operated from a central location could serve a majority of businesses better than a part-time service at the work place.

Although intake counselors are available and a procedure for handling alcohol, drug, and personal problem assessment and referral is in place, Memorial needs to develop a supervisory training program. A review of other employee assistance programs shows that supervisors at the work place need to be trained to spot individuals who have performance problems. The supervisors need to understand that their role is to refer these individuals to the employee assistance program rather than to act as counselors or diagnosticians. Also, employees need to be provided with information about alternative ways to reduce stress.

Thus, Memorial decides to focus on determining the costs of developing and implementing an employee assistance program and selling the service to a number of small local businesses. After determining all the costs—and paying particular attention to the cost of implementing and running the program—a price can be established.

Key Questions

To determine whether the hospital should continue with the planning process, a key hospital decision maker should answer a number of questions. If the answer to each question is yes, then the hospital should proceed to the next planning step. If the answer to any question is no, the hospital decision maker needs to investigate further or take action to change the answer to yes before proceeding with the planning process. These questions are:

- Do the hospital's resources and interests meet the health promotion needs of business and industry, or is the hospital willing to develop the resources needed? Yes _____ No _____
- Has a target market been clearly identified? Yes _____ No _____
- Can a program or service that appears to meet industry's needs be described? Yes _____ No _____
- Is that program compatible with hospital goals? Yes _____ No _____
- Have the cost estimates on all program elements been developed? Yes _____ No _____
- Has the hospital established a tentative price or price range for the service or program? Yes _____ No _____

Step 6. Sales Planning

Information from the prior five steps provides a basis for drafting a market-oriented sales plan, which should include financial projections. Now, armed with knowledge of the product or program and the businesses in the target market, the hospital can look at how the program will be sold.

Process

Up to this point, little consideration has been given to the process of selling. Is this service one that should be presented to the buyer by a salesperson? Is this a program that can be sold through direct mail advertising? Can this service be promoted through seminars, conventions, or meetings? If that is possible, the staff person becomes an organizer of meetings and an order taker. Would a group of businesses be willing to buy the service for the use of its members (associations, chambers of commerce, business coalitions)?

If so, fewer contacts need to be made in order to obtain a large volume of customers.

Sales Plan

Once the decision about the process is made, the next task is to establish a plan. If health promotion is the hospital's first program for business and industry, the first sales plan may be pure guesswork. However, even though it may appear to be based on little hard evidence, the initial plans should be put in writing. It is important to keep in mind that the sales plans can be altered after experience with the selling process.

The first thing to do is to list the companies in the target market that appear to be interested in the hospital's service, either because someone talked with them during the industry assessment or because they have a good, ongoing relationship with the hospital. The names of companies that are part of the target market but whose interest is unknown or who have no commitment to the hospital should be put on another list. The number of employees in each company should be included on these lists. Both lists will help in forecasting sales.

Next the hospital should plan how it will contact these companies. Will information about the service be sent in writing and followed up by a phone call? Another approach may be to invite company managers to attend a meeting.

The hospital needs to determine how much time it will need to make the initial contact and explain the program. It must also determine how long it will take to close the sale after the initial contact. From the client's perspective, the hospital is both offering a new service and acting as a new vendor. Thus, closing the sale may take much longer than was planned. The experiences of hospitals already providing such programs suggest that selling almost always takes longer than originally planned.

Once the precise method of contacting the customers has been determined, the hospital must estimate how many potential customers it can reach in a specified period. How many letters can be sent? How many calls can be made to customers who know about the proposed service? How many calls can be made to customers who are hearing about the proposed service for the first time? In making these estimates, it is important to be realistic about the time and energy involved.

Now is the time to try to estimate the number of buyers for the program. If the hospital is providing a single service, such as a program to prevent back injuries, it will have a higher ratio of buyers to sales calls. If it is offering a more complex service, such as an employee assistance program, it will not only take longer to get a decision to buy but the hospital may also have a lower ratio of calls to purchases.

Forecasting

The final step before actually committing funds to any program is to build a financial forecast that includes anticipated revenue and operating expenses. While there are many variations to this procedure, a basic profit and loss statement can be used to determine whether the forecast of sales applied against the costs of developing, selling, and operating the program will result in a profit and when that point will occur.

The hospital should develop an operating statement for the first three years of the program. This can be done by estimating when the first sale will occur and how much revenue it will generate and when subsequent sales will occur. This is the way to begin building the revenue portion of the statement.

There are three kinds of expenses that need to be accounted for: program development, program operation, and sales. Developmental costs will initially be heaviest at the beginning and may include such items as staff payroll, capital expense items, supplies, possible consultant expenses, and other variables related to the development of a specific service. Operating costs, which will begin just prior to implementing the program for the first client, will include both fixed and variable expenses such as payroll, facility costs (utilities and rent), maintenance and repair, equipment rental and service, contract labor, laboratory and medical costs, educational materials and publications, supplies, travel, and so forth. The third set of expenses, sales, will also be heaviest at the beginning of the program when printed and audiovisual promotional materials are developed as part of the sales process. Other sales expenses will include staff payroll, travel, and postage.

As in step 5, it would be wise to work closely with the hospital accountants in forecasting the proposed revenue and developmental expenses. They will be able to help establish costs for specific items, determine ways to account for depreciation and overhead chargebacks that the hospital may impose, and suggest the proper format to use in order to communicate effectively to others. The first forecast may not include all the costs of the program, either because they are unknown at the time or because the estimates were incorrect. Therefore, the forecast must be constantly revised as new information on costs becomes available. The forecast will serve as a resource in determining if a price change needs to be implemented and will be invaluable in estimating the costs of the next program the hospital may decide to develop.

What if the forecast is inaccurate and the costs are more than were anticipated? Even though the forecast is revised to reflect marketplace conditions, progress may be slower than expected because of an economic downturn, and the hospital's investment in this program may not be paying off as anticipated. At what point and based on what data will the hospital make the decision to withdraw this product line from the market? Although this is an unpleasant thought that dampens the enthusiasm for planning new programs, it is important that hospital management decide in advance how long the hospital will be able to carry a program or service that does not break even or create a profit. Hospitals have been accused, and perhaps justly, of seldom withdrawing services or programs that are not carrying their own weight. In planning, the hospital manager in charge of health promotion should determine how and when the decision to stop will be made.

Key Questions

To determine whether the hospital should continue with the planning process, a key hospital decision maker should answer a number of questions. If the answer to each question is yes, then the hospital should proceed with the development phase of the program. If the answer to any question is no, the hospital decision maker needs to investigate further or take action to change the answer to yes before proceeding. These questions are:

- Has the hospital selected a process for selling the service or program? Yes _____ No _____
- Has the hospital developed a plan for contacting customers? Yes _____ No _____
- Has the hospital developed an operating statement and profit and loss statement? Yes _____ No _____
- Is the hospital prepared to support the program until it becomes profitable? Yes _____ No _____
- Has the hospital set up criteria on which success or failure of this venture will be judged? Yes _____ No _____

Program Development, Evaluation, and Testing

At this point, the hospital has determined that providing health promotion services to business and industry does, indeed, fit with its mission and goals, and it has taken a client-oriented approach to determining what type of program has the best chance of success. To do this, the hospital has looked at the wants and needs of business and industry, at the resources within the hospital that will support the program, and at the obstacles that could stand in its way. After analyzing this information, the hospital has tentatively selected a program and target market and has probably begun to develop the new service. It has calculated potential costs, set a tentative price, planned a sales approach, and forecast sales.

Development

Now the hospital is ready to commit significant resources to fully developing the program or service to the point where it can be tested. Because there are many options regarding the particular type of service that the hospital may choose to develop, this publication is not designed to show you how to develop the specific content or components of an employee assistance program, an occupational health service, or a wellness, or life-style, program. However, regardless of which type of program is selected, it is vitally important that experts be used to develop and implement the specific service. For example, if an employee assistance program is being developed, experienced and qualified counselors and trainers should conduct the program. If the hospital is designing a fitness program, an exercise physiologist or other professional trained in physical fitness assessment and exercise should develop the program. If the hospital has decided to market behavior-changing activities, professionally trained health educators should develop the program.

Evaluation

At this point, the hospital must build a thorough evaluation component into any health promotion programs it is developing. Evaluation data will be invaluable as a future selling point in proving the value of the program to business and industry. Evaluation data also serve as an important factor at the point of sale to assure the prospective client that the hospital will provide the company with information on program outcomes. Businesses will want information documenting the implementation process as well as an assessment of the program staff's effectiveness. They will also look for data that document actual program results, measure participant and client satisfaction, and indicate the long-term effectiveness of health promotion programs. Because evaluation is such an important factor in establishing program credibility, the hospital may want to consider hiring outside experts or consultants to assist hospital staff in designing the evaluation component.

Testing

Once program components have been developed, they must be tested before being offered to business and industry. Testing the program or implementing it on a pilot basis provides an opportunity for the hospital to iron out any developmental difficulties and refine any problem areas. Equally important, it provides some valuable information about the program's effectiveness that can be used in selling the service to other businesses and industries.

The hospital should give serious consideration to providing the program to its own employees before attempting to sell it. Conducting the program for the hospital staff, even though they may be the toughest and most critical audience, will provide necessary experience and add greatly to the hospital's credibility in selling the program. Business and industry are much more likely to consider buying an employee health program from a supplier that has demonstrated its faith in the service by offering it to its own employees. Furthermore, the hospital should consider its responsibility to its own employees. If the institution is committed to keeping employees in the community healthy, it is imperative that it begin by providing health promotion services for its own employees.

REFERENCES

1. U.S. Department of Health, Education and Welfare. *Healthy People: The Surgeon General's Report on Health Promotion and Disease Prevention.* Washington, DC: HEW, 1979.
2. American Hospital Association. *The Hospital's Responsibility for Health Promotion.* Chicago: AHA, 1979.
3. MacStravic, Robin E. *Marketing Health Care.* Germantown, MD: Aspen Systems, 1977, p. 4.
4. Rotanz, Robert. Remarks at AHA conference entitled New Business Opportunities for Hospitals: Health Promotion Services for Local Industry, Orlando, FL, Feb. 23-25, 1981.
5. Gallagher, Michael J. Remarks at AHA conference entitled New Business Opportunities for Hospitals: Health Promotion Services for Local Industry, Orlando, FL, Feb. 23-25, 1981.

Chapter 5

Impact of Health Promotion
on Hospital and Business Environments

It is relatively easy to plan a health promotion program on paper. It is not easy to predict how flowcharts and planning documents will affect individuals. This is especially true of health promotion, which encompasses new ideas and programs and new ways of looking at life and health and creates new demands on both program staff and participants. Health promotion programs introduce many changes into the hospital organization. They may require a major refocus in the hospital's outlook: from illness to health, from prescriptions for patients to advice for clients, and from a not-for-profit orientation to a for-profit orientation.

This chapter describes what is likely to happen as a result of developing health promotion programs at the work site. It focuses on the impact of health promotion programs in three areas: the *hospital,* which provides the new health promotion program or service; the *employer,* who buys programs or services; and the *administrator or manager,* who directs the program or service.

Impact on the Hospital

Hospital management and governance must do the necessary groundwork before moving directly into program implementation. Changes that last occur slowly. The hospital must expend the necessary time and effort to determine how a health promotion program can serve its institutional goals. As discussed in chapter 2, the hospital must assess its expectations before venturing into the health promotion arena. If the hospital's governing board does not determine why it is getting into the health promotion business, the individuals responsible for program development will have difficulty explaining the programs, justifying the budget internally, and selling the services to business and industry.

Some board members, executive staff, and others will not be able to accept an for-profit operation. It is ironic, but not unusual, for a hospital board composed of businessmen who are making profits in their businesses every day to balk at selling profit-making services to local employers. Many boards may not readily accept the reality of a so-called charitable institution making money. Therefore, the hospital administrator must be prepared to marshal the arguments for generating profits: lack of third-party reimbursement, value of the services provided, and need to develop new, non-patient-care revenue sources to supplement the hospital's other patient-care services, and so forth.

Budget negotiations may create dissension among other departments in the hospital that believe they have a better claim to any money that is allocated to health promotion. If the hospital has not laid the groundwork for health promotion programs with the board of trustees and other key persons, it will not be able to avoid hostility toward the program or respond to questions like these: "How can you spend scarce resources on anything other than patient care?" "How can you ask for a marketing specialist or an administrator to run this new program when we desperately need another coronary care nurse?" "I've been begging for more lab space for three years. How can you say your project has a better claim than mine?" If the hospital can demonstrate the ways in which health promotion fulfills institutional objectives and fits into the hospital's long-range plans, it will be in a more advantageous bargaining position to obtain scarce resources.

Areas of support and opposition, and the strength of each, may be unexpected. A conservative member of the medical staff may be the staunchest supporter of a health promotion program, or conversely a usually docile trustee may insist that hospitals should be concerned solely with caring for the sick. It is not always possible to determine who will be a supporter or an adversary on the basis of a staff member's previous reaction to other newly initiated programs. Health promotion is different. One useful indicator, however, comes from the literature on innovation. It states that, in general, one-third of the persons the hospital wishes to influence will immediately see the wisdom of the plan and be willing to give some measure of support to it. Another third will have doubts but will change their minds as they begin to see positive results. And the final third will exhibit symptoms of opposition, from foot-dragging to outright sabotage, and will prove impossible to convert no matter how successful and accepted the health promotion program becomes. The hospital should spend its time and efforts on the first two-thirds. Universal agreement, like infinity, is unattainable.

Supporters of the program will want to move at a pace that is too fast for the hospital's support system. Those who are making the decision about health promotion must understand that it is crucial to take the time to gain support, line up resources, field-test and market-test services, and ensure that all the necessary persons are fully involved and committed. The decision maker must also determine whether present staff have the necessary interest, time, and capability to handle the increased demands and volume of activity created by a new program. The hospital also needs to assess its existing facilities and present service capabilities in terms of providing a greater volume and diversity of services. To succeed in enrolling business and industrial clients, the hospital needs a program that is verifiably well designed, of high quality, and ready for implementation.

Some hospital staff may interpret the health promotion program as a negative statement about past and current practices. Changes may be interpreted as criticism. It may be difficult for some health care professionals to recognize that programs and services must be adjusted to suit the concerns of the client. A hypothetical example is a nutritionist who has been successfully presenting in-service lectures on nutrition to groups of nurses for several years. Now the nutritionist is asked to change the program to suit the needs of a group of employees in a weight control class, to avoid lecturing, and to provide recipes. The nutritionist may need help in recognizing that the lectures, slides, and previous educational approach must be modified for nonprofessionals. Asking for these changes is not a criticism of past performance but a compliment to the professional who is seen as capable of making the adaptation.

Health promotion programs may encounter resistance from the medical staff. It is important to involve the medical staff early in the program-planning stages. If the hospital has decided exactly why it needs them and what it wants from them, this may not be difficult. For example, does it want to:

- Secure clinical confirmation of what it is planning to do? To get physican endorsement, it may be necessary to assist physicians in building their knowledge about health promotion and the concepts of preventive medicine. It may also be helpful to reassure them that the hospital program has no intention of competing with physicians' services.
- Encourage them to participate in planning and implementing the program? This is probably much harder to do, because physicians are not trained in these skills. The hospital should be specific about the roles and duties it would like physicians to fulfill.
- Obtain physician support or at least neutrality? The hospital may not need the active participation of the entire medical staff, but it cannot afford to have the physicians against the program. One approach is to form a medical advisory group for hospital health promotion activities. The purpose of this group is to discuss any objections and get physicians to participate in the planning process. Key physician leaders

should be consulted, and the hospital should listen carefully to physicians' advice and criticism. They have firsthand experience in dealing with future program participants. It is also important to provide the medical staff with regular follow-up reports once the program moves into operation, especially if physicians have been apprehensive about its development and its impact on their practices. The hospital should also identify physicians who will accept referrals when problems needing medical treatment are found among employees using health promotion services.

If the hospital does not begin health promotion programming with its own employees, the hospital will certainly hear from them. Many in the health promotion field believe that it is immoral to offer programs to outside clients and ignore the hospital's own employees. Employees may feel the same way. Providing in-house health promotion services is an excellent way to gain support from within and increase the hospital's credibility with potential clients. Business and industry may wonder how sincere the hospital's commitment to health promotion is if it has not bothered to set up a program for its own employees. Conversely, a potential client who is dubious about health promotion could be won over by seeing a successful program in action.

Developing a health promotion program may increase the hospital staff's involvement in patient education needs and create greater interest and demand for additional patient education resources. Changes may occur in the way patient care is delivered in the hospital as a result of large-scale involvement in health promotion. Exposure to health promotion activities may change the attitudes of some staff from nonbelievers to active participants in health education efforts. This may result in the medical staff placing greater emphasis on patient education efforts and requesting new educational materials and services. However, there is also a danger of the reverse happening, that is, a loss of interest in educating patients in favor of more exciting work-site programs.

Impact on the Employer

Health promotion programs also introduce changes into the companies that are the hospital's corporate clients. These programs are new "people systems" that affect employees and management as do such other people systems as salary administration, benefits, productivity programs, and organizational development. Clients must find ways to cope with the new ideas that the hospital is suggesting and deal with the impact on their organizations.

Health promotion programs will have wider repercussions than employers anticipate. It is a common experience for these programs to cause changes in the work place that seem to have nothing to do with health promotion. This is especially true of programs that stress wellness and life-style changes, which have a more direct effect on employee beliefs and attitudes than programs that are purchased for management purposes, that is, occupational health services such as safety inspections for compliance with regulations of the Occupational Safety and Health Administration (OSHA).

When employees learn to take responsibility for making decisions in one area of their lives in which they had previously been passive, they may become more assertive in changing other areas of their lives as well. It is possible that companies may find their employees less malleable, less acquiescent, and more inclined to question corporate expectations and policies. Employees may increase pressure on management to bring employees into the decision-making process in such areas as safety measures, working conditions, and benefit packages. Unions are likely to favor the increased assertiveness and involvement on the part of employees. However, management may be less enthusiastic.

Employers will thank you for letting them know in advance the spinoffs that can be expected as a result of implementing specific health promotion activities. Employer activities and policies may elicit the following reactions from employees:

- *Smoking cessation.* Employees who do not smoke may request that the employer establish no-smoking rules for organizational meetings, designate restricted smoking areas, and prohibit the sale of cigarettes. Conversely, smokers may react violently if they view the employer's actions to discourage smoking as an infringement of their individual rights.
- *Nutrition and weight control.* Employees may initiate suggestions regarding vending machine content, cafeteria menus, and amount of time allowed for the lunch break.
- *Exercise and fitness.* Employees may demand that the employer provide appropriate space and facilities, showers, dress code revisions, and time for employees to participate during the workday.
- *Safety.* Employees' concerns about exposure to hazardous substances at the work place and dangerous work practices or requirements may lead to requests for more stringent safety procedures and practices or requests for transfer to less hazardous work areas.
- *Life-style.* Employees may question present benefits and health insurance coverage and may request health pay instead of sick pay, time off for courses and activities, tuition reimbursement, and flexible hours.
- *Stress management.* Employees may demand changes in company norms and job pressures and ask for support from employee assistance programs.

Even the best-laid plans fail to meet all contingencies. If questions arise, who will handle them? The first protection against the unexpected is to decide why the hospital and the client are introducing the program. Some reasons may be to avoid government intervention, reduce turnover and absenteeism, or improve employee morale. Once the program's purpose in a specific business setting is understood, the hospital will be able to advise its client on how best to use its services. Implementation of the program must also be viewed from the client's perspective. How much time will be required from the business's staff to get the programs started? How will activities be conducted? Who will handle complaints and problems? It is important to appoint a program coordinator at the client site who can act as a liaison with the hospital in dealing with operational problems as they arise or, preferably, in advance. For example, someone in the business organization will need to assist the hospital in scheduling activities, contacting potential program participants, and monitoring employee satisfaction. It is also necessary to plan for backup arrangements within the hospital to maintain flexibility in responding to client needs.

Management's involvement and support for health promotion must be clearly communicated to employees by the way the program is structured. Access to services and availability of activities is a clear statement of the backing and commitment of management. Cost, scheduling, and access to and availability of services and facilities will all affect employees' involvement and participation in health promotion programs. Program planning must begin with firm management decisions concerning the following areas:

- *Eligibility.* Is the program offered to all employees or management only? Are programs offered on a voluntary or compulsory basis? Are there eligibility requirements to participate in specific activities?
- *Costs.* How much financial support will the program receive? Is the client prepared to commit additional resources, if necessary, to health promotion as the program develops? Does the budget provide for both additional program staff as well as adequate clerical staff to keep track of program activities and data? Will programs be provided to employees as a free benefit to encourage participation, or will employees be asked to pay for some classes or services to help ensure employee commitment?
- *Incentives.* Does the budget include money for incentives to encourage employee participation? What incentives will be both acceptable to management and attractive to employees: direct cash payments, class fee reimbursement, free buttons or T-shirts, subsidized healthy cafeteria menu selections, free enrollment or reduced membership fees at local health and fitness clubs, extra paid time off? Are incentives structured to appeal to the target employee population?
- *Scheduling.* Will testing programs, fitness activities, and educational classes be conducted during the workday, before or after work hours,

or on split-time (one half during the employee's personal time and one-half during the workday)? Are a majority of employees tied to commuter schedules that deter them from participating in programs before or after work hours? Are employees willing to use personal time during lunch hours to participate in ongoing health activities? Is the employer willing to offer flextime arrangements to create greater access to program activities? Will program activities need to be scheduled for different work shifts?

- *Access.* Are programs and facilities conducted at the employer site or at the hospital? If programs are conducted away from the business, how far will employees have to travel to participate? Is adequate space available at the work site to conduct a variety of programs? If fitness activities are conducted, do employees have access to shower and changing facilities?

Follow existing company norms and communication procedures in announcing and implementing health promotion programs. New employee health promotion activities should be introduced through the same means used to announce other employee programs, whether this be in the company newsletter, at managers' meetings, or at social gatherings. In general, the larger the company, the higher the value placed on following accepted internal communication procedures. If the hospital is being denied access to the usual employee communication media, there may be internal opposition to the health promotion program or, at the very least, apathy.

Impact on the Program Administrator

Because health promotion is a different kind of medical program, the individuals responsible for program development may notice differences in their professional life once they take charge of a hospital's health promotion service. The person who is identified with the program will be seen as an instant expert in all areas of health. That person may have to field questions such as "Why is it that when I jog, I get this funny little pain in my heel?" Clients may even seek medical consultation from the person, whether or not he or she has any medical training. They may also not be hesitant to point out that individual's own health shortcomings. If he or she is a smoker, obviously overweight, in poor physical condition, or a junk food junkie, he or she will certainly hear about it.

The person involved with the health promotion program may have to deal with some uncomfortable issues. It is not unusual to discover that companies are deliberately covering up unhealthy working conditions. Some firms will knowingly subject employees to an unhealthy amount of stress, even if there are other ways to achieve the same level of productivity. The person administering the program may come to believe that health promotion raises moral issues that must be addressed and that may affect the hospital's interest in continuing to serve certain clients.

A program administrator who has been in a care-giver role, such as a physician, nurse, or therapist, must make a shift in the way that he or she practices: from prescriber to adviser, from lecturer to teacher, from encouraging a patient to be compliant and dependent to helping a client achieve independence.

The program administrator will find that he or she stands out in the community. He or she may be criticized by some and will definitely be questioned about health promotion. However, it is to be hoped that he or she will also be recognized as someone who is performing a real and worthwhile service.

Chapter 6
Six Success Stories

Although health promotion is a relatively new concept, some hospitals have been providing health promotion services at the work place for several years. This chapter highlights the experiences and recommendations of six hospitals that have successfully developed and marketed health promotion programs to local business and industry. Each of the three major categories of health promotion programs, employee assistance, occupational health, and wellness, or life-style, is represented in these case studies.

- Case study 1, which describes an employee assistance program, is based on information provided by Paula Bills, manager, Priority Systems for Employee Assistance, Overlook Hospital, Summit, New Jersey.
- Case study 2, which describes a wellness, or life-style, program, is based on information provided by Stephen D. Gelineau, assistant administrator, Union Hospital, Lynn, Massachusetts.
- Case study 3, which also describes a wellness, or life-style, program, is based on information provided by Donald W. Zeigler, director, Good Health Program, Skokie Valley Community Hospital, Skokie, Illinois.
- Case study 4, which describes an occupational health program, is based on information provided by Michael J. Gallagher, vice-president of operations, Swedish American Hospital, Rockford, Illinois.
- Case study 5, which also describes an occupational health program, is based on information provided by David J. Heritage, director, Occupational Health Service, Franklin County Hospital, Greenfield, Massachusetts.
- Case study 6, which describes a comprehensive program, is based on

information provided by Linda Hawes Clever, M.D., chairman, Department of Occupational Health, Presbyterian Hospital of Pacific Medical Center, San Francisco, California.

Additional information on the experiences of 150 hospitals that have developed and marketed health promotion programs to business and industry is included in the survey described in appendix A. The hospitals participating in the survey were those hospitals that sent representatives to the conferences on which this publication is based.

Case Study 1. Employee Assistance Program at Overlook Hospital

Overlook Hospital is a 550-bed teaching hospital located in Summit, New Jersey, a suburban community of New York City. The employee assistance program at Overlook Hospital provides services for more than 18,000 employees in 14 businesses. These businesses are primarily health-related industries and insurance companies that employ mostly white-collar workers. They tend to be economically stable businesses that already provide substantial benefit packages to their employees.

Objectives

The employee assistance program at Overlook Hospital was designed to meet three primary objectives:
- Respond to the business community's request for emergency services, counseling, and referral resources for employees whose personal problems were affecting their on-the-job performance
- Make the hospital a comprehensive and total resource for all community health care needs
- Provide a self-sustaining and revenue-producing program

Components

Overlook Hospital provides the following services to businesses that contract for services:
- Assistance in organizational policy and procedure development, including consultation on development of supervisory training guidelines
- Assistance in developing all employee promotional materials, such as brochures and posters
- Employee orientation sessions about the employee assistance program
- Supervisor training sessions
- Counseling, which involves assessment of individual employees who are referred to the program or self-referred for identification of problems, consultation with employees on their specific problems, and their referral

to other counseling or follow-up programs as necessary
- Training in-house coordinators to handle problems in program logistics at the work site
- Quarterly reports, which include anonymous information about demographics and data on employees who have used the program

Development

The program as initially conceived was designed to help employers identify employees with alcohol problems. The hospital applied for and was awarded a grant from the National Institute of Alcohol Abuse and Alcoholism (NIAAA) to conduct a demonstration project for two large local employers, Bell Laboratories and Ciba-Geigy Pharmaceutical Company, and for the employees of the hospital. Today, the hospital's employee assistance program, called Priority Systems for Employee Assistance, deals with all types of personal problems, such as family and marital stress or alcohol or drug abuse.

A major impetus in developing the program was provided by the medical director of the Department of Community Health. The medical director brought together a planning committee, which consisted of persons from the community health, finance, and personnel departments and members of the hospital's Professional Advisory Committee.

The medical director sent a memo to all hospital medical staff members asking them if they were interested in serving on an advisory committee to develop an employee assistance program. Five physicians indicated an interest in serving on this planning committee. Other physicians were kept informed of program developments but played no active role.

Development of the program took one year, from the start of planning to the time the first business client was contacted.

Overlook Hospital initially offered the program to its own employees before going to businesses. At first, hospital employees were skeptical about the confidentiality of a program that was conducted in-house, but now they accept it. The number of hospital employees using the program has increased from 3 to 5 percent annually.

The program is staffed by a manager, assistant manager, and four counselors. The hospital has renovated a house on the hospital grounds for the program and its staff.

Marketing Strategy

Members of the hospital's board of trustees helped to promote the employee assistance program to local business contacts.

Most businesses that Overlook Hospital is presently working with are large companies that contracted for program services because they saw the program as an employee benefit. Overlook is now contacting smaller companies that have fewer dollars to spend on benefits and are consequently looking for cost-effective ways to provide benefits to employees. The service is also sold as a management tool to assist employees with job performance problems.

The hospital has moved from an intensive marketing development approach to a strong sales approach now that the program is fully developed. It has hired the services of an advertising agency and a sales representative to assist in selling and promoting the program. The advertising agency is helping the hospital develop a direct mail campaign, a public relations approach, and a radio, television, and print media campaign.

Funding and Fees

Initially the program received grant funding with supplemental funding from the hospital. Now the program is self-sustaining from revenue generated. The hospital is at present considering the establishment of a self-sufficient, investor-owned corporation to operate the program.

Fees are based on program costs, as determined by volume of service and projected expenses. Businesses are charged on a per capita basis ($20 for each employee in the organization whether or not the employee actually uses the program).

Strategies for Success

Paula Bills, manager of Priority Systems, suggests that hospitals interested in starting such a program should consider the following points:
- The hospital should *do careful planning and market research* so that the program is organized to meet specific business and industry needs.
- The hospital should *be realistic in determining program costs* and know what local business and industry are willing to invest for a program that does not immediately pay for itself.

Case Study 2. Life-Style Program at Union Hospital

Union Hospital is a fully accredited and licensed 210-bed community health care center providing comprehensive diagnostic and therapeutic medical, surgical, and mental health services to the citizens of Greater Lynn and portions of the Massachusetts North Shore. Union is located in Lynn, a coastal community approximately 12 miles northeast of Boston.

The hospital became active in health education during 1974, when, after formal endorsement by its board of trustees, it first offered programs to the community. Since then, approximately 30,000 residents have attended one of the 300 programs that have been offered on a wide range of subjects, such as nutrition, smoking cessation, arthritis, heart disease, stress management, depression, diabetes, aerobic exercise, cancer, and home emergencies. Most of these programs are offered at the hospital or community sites on weekday evenings at low cost, and some are still free.

Components

In 1979, the hospital more formally organized its health education efforts by establishing the North Shore Institute of Health. Today, the institute is a regional health promotion and disease prevention service offering a wide variety of programs for hospitals, schools, businesses, industries, and the community. The institute's efforts toward business and industry are centered around a portfolio of programs called Health Development Services. These programs are designed for presentation to employees at the work site. They are on such subjects as stress management, alcoholism, physical fitness and exercise, smoking cessation, nutrition and weight control, and body mechanics. The hospital also offers business and industry an employee assistance program and expects to add a comprehensive occupational health service during 1982 or 1983.

Development

The Health Development Service portfolio was created by a planning committee that included the hospital's administrator, assistant administrator, and director of marketing; the director of the Greater Lynn Community Mental Health Center; and the staff director and the medical director of the North Shore Institute of Health. Additionally, the market research included discussions with selected business and industry leaders as well as business round tables, at which the subject of the health promotion and disease prevention needs in business and industry were discussed over lunch. Union Hospital's market research also included a careful study of the literature on these types of programs. According to hospital assistant administrator Stephen D. Gelineau, "We believe the research process is an ongoing function that must continually monitor the marketplace for changes in needs, wants, or perceptions." As a result, the hospital still carries on a modified version of the market research process described above.

During the program planning stages, the effort received strong support from all the hospital's internal groups: trustees, medical staff, administration, and employees. Gelineau attributes this to the institution's strong historic orientation to community service. "In addition," he said, "the hospital was already offering similar programs to the community, so it wasn't a new concept."

As mentioned earlier, Health Development Services are conducted at the work site. The decision to provide the programs in this way was made because space at the hospital was limited and because the convenience of programs based at the work site was an attractive selling point for the employer.

Fees

Program fees are determined by calculating all direct and indirect expenses associated with a given service (including overhead and promotional expenses) and then adding an appropriate markup, usually 20 percent. The programs may be purchased in individual components or as a total package at a reduced price.

Clients

Since the inception of its business and industry effort, Union has provided programs and services to approximately 75 companies and organizations. Client companies vary in size from 30 to more than 1,000 employees and include a creamery, an auto dealership, a meat company, and other manufacturing, industrial, and high-technology concerns. The most popular programs are those on stress management and alcoholism. The employee assistance program is also a popular service.

Strategies for Success

Key factors that can influence a hospital's ability to develop this type of effort include:

- *Staff.* Someone who can shoulder full responsibility for both the management and coordination of the program will be needed. This person must be at a recognized supervisory level. Furthermore, a determination must be made as to which staff members in the hospital are capable of delivering these types of services.
- *Services.* Within the broad spectrum of health promotion and disease prevention, a determination must be made as to which programs can be effectively and efficiently delivered and which of these are needed by business and industry. This implies careful and thorough market research.
- *Facilities.* In Union's case, hospital meeting space was so limited that a program that would be delivered at the work site was a virtual requirement. Hospitals with attractive, convenient, and available meeting locations may prefer to use their own facilities, although employers are known to like the convenience of work-site programs.
- *Cost.* Start-up costs are inevitable and a calculated risk. The hospital must be prepared for initial losses that occur during early program implementation. The hospital must also determine how much money it can afford to lose, using a worst-case situation.

- *Time.* Most programs need two to three (and sometimes more) years to break even. Can the hospital wait that long? Also, do the hospital professionals who have been selected to deliver these programs have enough time to deliver them? Do the employees of the business or industry have enough time to participate? What about before-work or after-work programs? What about second, third, or weekend shift availability of the hospital staff?
- *Reputation.* While the focus is usually on how the new program might enhance the hospital's future reputation, it is also true that the hospital's current reputation can hinder acceptance of the program. Furthermore, whereas a hospital might have an excellent reputation within its immediate service area, it might be completely unknown to some of the business and industry to which it seeks to sell its programs.

Finally, Gelineau's encouragement to other hospitals developing health promotion programs for industry is: "Don't be afraid to experiment and innovate. Nobody has written the last word in this area yet."

Case Study 3. Life-Style Program at Skokie Valley Community Hospital

Skokie Valley Community Hospital is a 284-bed facility located northwest of Chicago in suburban Skokie, Illinois. The business community in its service area is quite diverse and includes large corporate headquarters, service industries, small businesses, and heavy and light manufacturing.

Objectives

Skokie Valley Community Hospital developed its Good Health Program in 1978 as a result of a board of trustees policy decision to develop a model hospital primary prevention and life-style program that would also demonstrate private sector initiative in cutting medical care costs through disease prevention. Unlike most hospitals, Skokie Valley did not view the Good Health Program as a profit center. However, the trustees did hope that the program would become self-sustaining within several years and made a decision to continue the program only if it demonstrated positive life-style changes in a substantial number of participants.

Components

The Good Health Program offers several packages for employee groups. The program has three components: (1) a *life-style assessment,* during which participants learn the extent to which their current behaviors are creating health hazards, (2) in-depth *health promotion workshops* aimed at helping individuals change unhealthy behaviors, and (3) *periodic program follow up and evaluation.* All of these components are offered at the work site.

The life-style assessment, the most extensive component offered by the Good Health Program, consists of a computerized health risk assessment (HRA), a life-style physical screening, and a results session. Employees complete a questionnaire that assesses their personal and family medical history and individual life-style practices. Employees then participate in a physical screening, which measures height, weight, skinfold (body fat), and blood pressure and includes tests for blood cholesterol (HDL) and urine sugar. Tests to screen for cancer of the colon and for glaucoma are given to individuals over a specific age. Individuals also participate in a submaximal step test to measure their fitness levels. The questionnaire data and the results of the clinical tests are then processed by computer.

Participants receive individualized, confidential reports, which are returned and explained during a group results session. Individuals who have abnormal test results are referred to their private physicians for further consultation or treatment. In some situations, the results session may be enlarged to serve as a single educational session (lasting 1-1/2 hours) for groups unable to participate in more extensive educational programs. Generally, however, the health promotion activities consist of overview sessions ranging in number from 5 to 16 sessions on specific topics, such as aerobics fitness, to help participants change unhealthy behaviors and reduce their risk of disease or illnesses. Educational sessions are on these topics: nutrition, weight control, stress management, exercise, smoking cessation, and cancer prevention and self-examination.

Evaluation has been a key program component. Accordingly, quantitative process and impact evaluation measures were set up to demonstrate statistically valid behavior changes among participants who repeat the health risk assessment after one year.

Development

When Skokie Valley's trustees decided to move into the health promotion field, they created a separate auxiliary, the Good Health Board of Directors, to vividly demonstrate the priority status of the pilot project. Its members include the chairman of the board of trustees, the president of the medical staff, the hospital's chief executive officer, and several other health care professionals. This high-level membership demonstrated hospital interest and has been an asset with area employers.

A basic decision was to design a program of the highest quality. This resulted in a program best suited for the largest employers. The hospital's initial market assessment zeroed in on employee groups of 250 or more, although variations of the program now make services practical for groups of fewer than 50 persons.

The hospital began rapid program development in May 1978. In a six-month time span, the program director surveyed local industry and other existing programs (although few existed in that year), assessed the hospital's resources, and drafted a program plan. A Fun Run and stop-smoking clinics for the community were sponsored to give the program visibility during the developmental phase.

By January 1979, program staff were hired to implement a pilot screening program and health education classes for the hospital's employees. Forty-six percent of the hospital's employees went through the program during a five-month period.

Program director Don Zeigler says the pilot program taught staff members several lessons: Flexibility is needed when providing programs to employees working in various locations. Once curricula are established, contracting educational services can be considered, though cautiously. In addition, the pilot experience showed that the expectations for the program were far too high because of the hospital's lack of experience, poor local economy, and slow acceptance of health promotion by employers, although the latter is improving.

Staffing and Implementation

The hospital has seven full-time employees to staff the Good Health Program. These include the program administrative director, an assistant director, a nutritionist, a smoking program coordinator, and one health educator/screening coordinator. An exercise physiologist is employed part-time. The program contracts with outside consultants to conduct stress management classes. Several part-time technicians and a part-time secretary provide additional program support.

All services are delivered at the work site. To reach the largest number of employees, assessment sessions can be scheduled before or after work hours, at lunch, and during all work shifts. The program staff tries to schedule health promotion workshops during the workday, but they have found that not all employers are willing to adjust workers' schedules. Most employers expect these activities to be carried out during employees' own time.

Funding

A board member secured start-up funding from a local foundation during the early development phase. Other grants were subsequently secured. The hospital board has approved program subsidies over the past three years, during which time program revenue was expected to build. Hospital support has been less than 0.5 percent of Skokie Valley Hospital's general operating revenue.

Fees

Employers are charged a uniform, per capita fee for each employee who participates in the HRA and screening program. A separate fee is charged for each group educational workshop:

- Stop Smoking Clinic (6 sessions of 1-1/2 hours each)
- Nutrition/Eating for Good Health (5 sessions of 1 hour each)
- Stress Management (5 sessions of 1 hour each)
- Weight Control (14 sessions of 45 minutes each)
- Introduction to Exercise (4 sessions of 1 hour each)
- Dance Fitness or Exercise for Good Health (12 sessions of 1 hour each)
- You Can Control Your Risk for Cancer (1 session of 45 minutes)

Most employers, at the hospital's suggestion, require employees to pay a portion of the program fees (from $10 to one-half of the program fee) to defray costs and ensure commitment to the program.

Clients

The Good Health Program is working with several large organizations. Its clients include Northwestern University (the largest, with 5,000 employees), the local high school district, and the corporate headquarters of Washington National Insurance Company, Brunswick Corporation, Allstate Insurance Company, and Quaker Oats Corporation. The hospital is currently redesigning elements of the Good Health Program to accommodate the needs of the small employer, for example, Baha'i National Center and several local police departments.

Strategies for Success

Zeigler believes that the following points are important in creating and maintaining a successful health promotion effort:

- The hospital should *keep physicians informed* of program development. Skokie Valley faced strong opposition from the medical staff. It softened this opposition by keeping physicians informed of program development and providing high-quality community programs to which physicians could refer patients. However, this did not eliminate opposition. Zeigler thinks that eliminating all opposition is unlikely; change will come about over time as the results of health promotion programs become more evident.
- The hospital should *be prepared to provide answers when potential clients ask for data* demonstrating that health promotion reduces premature deaths, illness, absenteeism, and insurance costs. Zeigler's response: "While all of the data are not in yet, we do know that the major causes of illness are largely linked to life-style. Prudence dictates that

training persons to alter life-styles in order to stay healthy will be less expensive than treating the individuals once they become ill. Also, healthy living is likely to increase productivity and longevity and offer a better quality of life. Further, unhealthy behaviors are identifiable and changeable, as shown in our results thus far." Fortunately, the literature demonstrating the effectiveness of health promotion is increasing, and so hospitals should keep looking at professional publications and local papers for evidence of the effectiveness of health promotion programs.

- The hospital *must make tough decisions about target market and pricing.* The Good Health Program, which was initiated during a time when few institutions had any experience in such programs, projected that a work force of at least 250 employees was necessary to produce enough volume to sustain the life-style screening and follow-up classes. Thus, it concentrated its initial marketing efforts on large employers. Anticipating large volumes, the hospital set low initial fees, which later had to be raised.
- The hospital should *decide whether components of the program will be offered separately.* Some, maybe most, companies will be interested only in certain aspects of the program or will not be able to budget enough the first year for the entire program. The hospital must decide how far it will compromise, based on quality and cost considerations.
- The hospital should *be flexible and creative* in its program offerings and schedulings, especially with factory, shift-work, and dispersed employee populations.
- The hospital should *be aware of changing economic conditions that may affect business decisions regarding health promotion.* Cost containment considerations, however, definitely favor prevention programs.
- The hospital should *demand a quality program and be willing to spend the time and money needed to achieve it.* The goal, where possible, should be to create a program that is effective in obtaining significant life-style changes. Otherwise, the hospital's efforts will be wasted, and the health promotion movement will be discredited.
- The hospital should *seek alternative means to pay for health promotion.*

Case Study 4. Occupational Health Program at Swedish American Hospital

Swedish American is a 421-bed teaching hospital in Rockford, Illinois. It is located in an urban area with a full range of business enterprises. The hospital has been involved in industrial medicine to some extent since 1930. However, it was not until 1977 that the hospital established a separate occupational health program.

Objectives

Swedish American Hospital developed its program to achieve the following goals:

- Respond to concerns expressed by existing business clients
- Take steps to reverse an emerging pattern of declining referrals of industrial injury cases to emergency and outpatient treatment departments
- Diversify from acute inpatient care to outpatient care
- Focus community attention on the hospital as a provider of high-quality, innovative care targeted to local needs.
- Realize a profit that could support other hospital services

Components

Occupational health offerings at Swedish American include:

- Physician-directed medical services, such as preemployment physical examinations, treatment of work-related injuries, and return-to-work disability evaluations
- Hearing conservation program
- Personnel evaluation and counseling services
- Occupational assessment services, including vocational and psychological testing for specific job functions
- Chronic pain clinic

Staffing

The hospital has expanded its occupational health services to include an employee assistance program, occupational health education, and a wellness, or life-style, program. All these programs are currently being marketed to employers in the community. In addition, an employer health care audit and other programs are currently being developed and tested for marketing in 1982.

It is the hospital's policy to deliver these services when and where the client wishes (most often at the work site). Implementing this policy requires a substantial staff, which includes a part-time medical director, full-time administrative director, part-time chronic-pain clinic medical director, consulting psychologist, two pain clinic nurses, two nurses to conduct screening and education programs, two clerical and billing employees, and an office manager. The program also requires the participation of many physicians in private practice.

Development

The administration of Swedish American Hospital took the lead in all program planning. Most market research was carried out by hospital staff, although a consultant was also retained.

The hospital assessed the needs of local business and industry in several ways:

- The hospital conducted an analysis of its own business ties to determine which employee groups used the hospital the most, which employers paid a significant portion of the hospital's revenue, and what type of services were used by the employee groups.
- The hospital also surveyed local business and industry during an 18-month period to assess their needs. Written questionnaires were distributed to more than 1,200 companies. The hospital then conducted 70 personal follow-up interviews with individual businesses who responded to the survey and indicated that they would like more information about programs that the hospital was developing.
- Local insurance carriers of interested businesses were contacted to get a precise picture of the company's occupational health service needs. The names of specific insurance companies and permission to contact them were obtained from the businesses during the market research interviews.
- Through direct contracts with the employers of various employee groups, the hospital compiled a list of occupational health services offered by competitive-investor-owned organizations.

After completing the assessment of needs and demands of local business and industry, the hospital then matched the unmet industrial needs to its own resources and strengths. Some existing hospital services, such as the examination and testing programs, could be readily offered to business and industry with little or no change. Other services, such as the pain clinic, psychological counseling services, and special screening programs, needed to be developed. However, in some cases, the hospital determined that it did not have the expertise or that it was not feasible to develop a particular program. The hospital then assumed the role of a broker by matching various employer needs to existing programs or health care services in the community, whether or not they were operated directly by Swedish American Hospital. For example, if an employer requests physical fitness programs or facilities, the hospital facilitates contracts with the local YMCA to provide fitness activities to the business.

To ensure physician acceptance, the hospital involved the medical staff in the program design process at an early stage. It also conducted the programs for hospital employees before soliciting clients.

Most start-up funds came from the operating budgets of the departments providing services. Because fees for the program were based on full cost recovery plus a minimum 8 percent margin, it was possible to plan for a breakeven point by the end of the second year of operation of a new program or service.

Swedish American Hospital provides services to approximately 150 industrial clients on a regular basis. The services most frequently requested are industrial environmental assessments, physical evaluations, and pain clinic referrals.

Strategies for Success

Swedish American's vice-president for operations, Michael J. Gallagher, recommends that hospitals focus on the following key factors to ensure program success:

- The hospital should *solve any internal problems* before presenting clients with a package of services. Examples of internal hospital problems that may need attention are emergency department waiting time, billing department capabilities, and coordination of diagnostic department services to efficiently serve a client's employees.
- One successful selling strategy is to *upgrade relationships and volume with existing client firms before presenting the program to new clients*. Existing clients are also the best initial market for new program components; current successes give the hospital credibility as it seeks to develop further services.
- The hospital must *plan on a minimum of six to nine months* to properly assess needs, design the program, initiate marketing, and sign up the first customer. At Swedish American, this process took 15 months.
- The hospital must *plan to spend money* before it makes money.
- *At least one person should be assigned* to the project full-time from the start to ensure program continuity and development.

Case Study 5. Occupational Health Program at Franklin County Public Hospital

Franklin County Public Hospital is a 162-bed, private, not-for-profit hospital in Greenfield, Massachusetts. It serves a primarily rural area that has some light manufacturing and industrial firms (plastics, paper, machine tool fabrication, small foundry operations, power companies). Most businesses in the area have an average of 130 employees and are thus too small to afford in-house health services.

Objectives

Franklin County Public Hospital focused on three primary objectives in developing its occupational health service program. First, the hospital had received several industrial requests for specific services and was therefore interested in addressing this community need. Second, it viewed the area of occupational health as an opportunity to maximize utilization of the hospital's outpatient services. A third objective was to generate new revenue. The program was planned to be self-sustaining, with a profit expected by the third or fourth year of operation.

Components

Franklin County offers business and industrial clients the following occupational health services:
- Preplacement and periodic health examinations
- Emergency treatment for industrial injuries and follow-up care
- Return-to-work examinations
- Workers' compensation evaluations
- Executive physical examinations
- Tests and laboratory work (hearing, pulmonary function, X rays) required by the Occupational Safety and Health Administration (OSHA)
- Employee assistance programs
- Health education programs

Development

Because Franklin County is a small hospital, program planning was conducted on an informal basis. Staff members who were primarily active in the planning process were the chief executive officer; vice-president for fiscal services; interested physicians; administrator of rehabilitation services, who became director of the program; marketing consultant brought in to survey local industry needs; and department heads most directly concerned with program services.

Once a decision to develop an occupational health service program was made, intrahospital communication became mor² formal. Meetings, orientation sessions, and discussion groups were held on a regular basis with all the service areas involved. The participation of the medical staff was actively solicited, and a concerted effort was made to keep its members informed from the start of planning.

Services are provided both at the hospital and at the work place. A mobile trailer is equipped to conduct many testing services at the work site. If an employee comes to the hospital for testing, individual services are performed by the appropriate departments.

During the early stages of the planning process, Franklin County discovered that the major components of the occupational health program were already in place and functioning. The hospital was operating a 24-hour emergency care service for industrial injuries. A number of departments were also already providing services that local business and industry needed. For example, the speech and hearing department performed audiometric testing, respiratory therapy conducted pulmonary function tests, radiology provided chest and back X rays, Health education provided first aid and cardiovascular pulmonary resuscitation training as well as consultation on diet and nutrition, and mental health services operated an employee assistance program unit and provided comprehensive inpatient and outpatient psychiatric care and alcohol abuse treatment.

Once these existing services were identified, the hospital began to develop a package of services to offer to industrial clients. Because the hospital already had experience in conducting these programs, it decided not to pilot test the program with its own employees or with a single prospective client before moving directly into marketing and sales. As a result, the hospital was able to sign its first industrial client only six months after initial program discussions began.

Program development is an ongoing process. Franklin County plans to put greater emphasis on life-style programs for its industrial clients and to offer their clients consultation on their insurance coverage and health benefit packages.

Staffing

The occupational health program staff includes a medical director, an administrative director, an occupational health nurse, and a secretary. Other hospital staff members function as backup personnel to provide clinical services so that the hospital can always meet client requests on a timely basis. In this way the hospital is able to maximize utilization of its existing personnel without having to hire new staff to provide program services.

Funding and Fees

Franklin County relied entirely on its operating resources to initiate and develop the program. Most services are provided on a fee-for-service basis. Program fees are regulated by the Massachusetts Rate Setting Commission, which requires the same charges for business and private customers. This means that there are standard rates for all one-time outpatient services, although in some cases the hospital can offer volume discounts (for example, mass testing programs) and capitated rates (for example, employee assistance programs).

Clients

Today, Franklin County provides occupational health services to some 35 industrial clients. The services that are most frequently requested are hearing testing, preplacement physicals, and employee assistance programs.

Strategies for Success

On the basis of the hospital's experience, program administrator David J. Heritage offers the following advice:

- In marketing a program, the hospital must *be professional* in its approach. It should maintain regular contact and visibility with prospective clients. Local chapters of industrial, employer, commercial, and safety organizations should be used to spread the word about the hospital's program. It is vital that the hospital listen to its clients and solicit their ideas. The hospital should offer no panaceas and make no promises that it cannot keep. It should sell cost-effectiveness whenever it can be demonstated. Most important, the hospital must *be flexible* in meeting its clients' needs.
- The hospital should *anticipate and plan for a negative reaction from the medical staff*. It is important to have an interested physician associated with the program so that he or she can articulate the program's objectives and purposes to peers.
- The hospital should *take stock of the services it currently offers*. The basic components of an occupational health service may already be in place. Wherever possible, it is better to use existing services and methods of operation than to develop new ones.
- Once the program has been marketed and publicized, the hospital should *get the program into operation quickly*. It is important not to lose momentum.

Case Study 6. Comprehensive Program at Pacific Medical Center

San Francisco's Pacific Medical Center is a health care complex that includes the 341-bed Presbyterian Hospital, the 129-bed Garden Sullivan Hospital, and the Institute of Medical Sciences, a research arm of the institution. The existence of multiple resources led the center to believe that it was in a good position to provide employee health services to the large and diversified business community of the metropolitan area, and in 1977 it inaugurated the first such program on the West Coast.

Objectives

Pacific Medical Center did not experience much opposition from physicians in developing services for business and industry. In fact, key medical leaders provided the interest and impetus for the program and carried it through necessary changes in the bylaws of the center. The goals for the program were to fill an unmet need for health care, attract new persons to the hospital's sphere of influence, and continue the hospital's reputation for innovation.

Components

Pacific Medical Center began its program with the establishment of the Department of Occupational Health, and its program still bears that title. Over the years, however, the program has expanded to encompass life-style and employee assistance components. Services offered include:

- Development of medical surveillance programs
- Psychiatric crisis intervention and long-term counseling
- Emergency care
- Treatment of work-related injuries
- Assistance complying with regulations of the Occupational Safety and Health Administration (OSHA) and in meeting other environmental regulations at the work place
- Disability evaluation, including determination of the relationship of the condition to the work place
- Preplacement and periodic physical history and examinations
- Stress management
- Fitness counseling
- Smoking cessation
- Nutritional counseling
- Cardiopulmonary resuscitation and Heimlich maneuver instruction
- Pain evaluation and treatment

The program has a medical director, but it relies less on its own department staff than on referrals to other areas of the hospital, for example, physiotherapy, vocational rehabilitation, alcoholism treatment, laboratory services, emergency department, and continuing education. Services are delivered both at the hospital, which renovated some space especially for this purpose, and at the work site.

Development

The hospital set up a planning committee consisting of the chairmen of the departments of medicine and psychiatry, members of the board of trustees, and representatives from big business. The eventual purchasers of occupational health and health promotion services were thus involved directly in the entire development process, rather than simply being consulted about their needs. Pacific Medical Center had a partial market survey carried out by a consulting firm.

The hospital developed an extensive and comprehensive health program for its own employees. This was crucial to developing efficient and effective services for several reasons: hospital workers face serious health hazards, the hospital could "fine tune" the program before it was offered to the public, and the hospital showed clients that it practiced what it preached.

From the beginning, the program provided a "one phone call" service for business and industry so that clients could contact the Department of Occupational Health for assistance with all of their employee health problems. The hospital has designed one-of-a-kind programs to meet an individual client's specific needs. Pacific Medical Center's special programs have included:

- Administering gamma globulin shots to office workers exposed to hepatitis
- Teaching cardiopulmonary resuscitation to employees of accounting and construction firms
- Providing health education for workers exposed to lead
- Evaluating companies' emergency planning, from first-aid kits to earthquake preparedness

Strategies for Success

Linda Hawes Clever, M.D., medical director of the Department of Occupational Health, offers the following suggestions:

- The hospital should *be surveyed to determine what limitations exist* in terms of scheduling, volume, billing, staff opposition, and space. Addressing these problems before becoming operational is crucial to success.
- The hospital must *focus on marketing analysis and promotion.* This was one of the weak areas at Pacific Medical Center, and the hospital has since learned to identify those business and labor leaders who are already interested in health promotion. For the others, the hospital found that education must precede selling. Some of the methods used to inform corporate and union representatives about the hospital and its purposes are special luncheons, slide shows, and personal presentations by hospital department chairmen.

Appendix A

Survey of Conference Participants

In December 1981, AHA's Center for Health Promotion distributed a survey to 566 individuals who had participated in past sessions of the conference "New Business Opportunities for Hospitals: Health Promotion Services for Local Industry." The conference was first conducted in 1979, and three more sessions were held during 1980-81. The survey was conducted to determine how many hospitals that sent representatives to the conferences were at present involved in marketing health promotion programs to business and industry and to determine the extent and nature of the hospitals' activities in this area.

Because the number of hospitals that participated in the survey is relatively small, the data cannot be accepted as a randomly selected representative of the hospital field in general. However, these responses can be viewed as the first data summarizing hospitals' experiences in developing and marketing health promotion services for business and industry and can provide useful information to other institutions who are providing similar services.

Total Responses

A total of 150 hospitals responded to the survey. Of the total respondents:
- 40 percent (58 hospitals) reported they were actively marketing and conducting health promotion services for business and industry and had business clients
- 55 percent (84 hospitals) reported that they were not at present marketing health promotion services, although many said that they anticipated developing programs in the near future or were in the preliminary market research and planning stages of program development

- 5 percent (8 survey respondents) were nonhospital conference participants

Respondent Demographics

The hospitals that responded to the survey were primarily community not-for-profit hospitals located in urban or suburban areas. The majority of these hospitals had between 200 and 400 beds. The second largest category of respondents was hospitals having between 500 and 1,000 beds.

Type of Programs

Of the 58 hospitals that indicated they were marketing health promotion programs to industry:
- 24 hospitals reported that they were marketing employee assistance programs
- 43 hospitals reported they were marketing occupational health services
- 47 hospitals reported they were marketing wellness, or life-style, programs

Program Development

The individual(s) or areas within the hospital identified as being primarily responsible for health promotion program development, in order of frequency of response, were:
- Administrator
- Health education or community relations department
- Planning department

Less frequently mentioned were physicians and boards of trustees.

The most common reasons for program development, in order of frequency of response, were:
- Improve hospital's public image
- Build good relationships with local businesses
- Improve health of the community
- Respond to industry requests
- Increase non-patient-care revenues
- Increase inpatient referrals

All six of these reasons were cited by almost all of the respondents.

Market Research

Two-thirds of the hospitals that responded to the survey indicated that they had conducted a market survey to determine what programs or services were needed by the business community.

The methods that the respondents most frequently used in their survey

of business and industry, in order of frequency of response, were:
- Personal interviews
- Written questionnaires
- Telephone interviews

The majority of hospitals (32) that conducted market research surveys used internal staff to conduct the market survey; 11 hospitals used market research specialists.

The majority of hospitals contacted either fewer than 25 or more than 100 businesses in their market survey.

One-half of the respondents indicated that they received less than 25-percent response rate to the market survey. Most of the remaining hospitals indicated that they received a 100-percent response.

The type of business and industry to which hospitals most often marketed health promotion programs was listed according to frequency of response:
- Small businesses with fewer than 200 employees
- Large corporations
- Service industries and heavy manufacturers

Internal Development

Slightly more than half of the respondents indicated they had used a planning committee to develop health promotion programs. The key individuals most frequently identified by hospitals as participating on the planning committee were:
- Administrators
- Physicians
- Health educators

Less frequently mentioned were planners, public relations staff, trustees, and financial staff. Other individuals occasionally mentioned as planning committee participants were community and business group representatives, nurses, personnel department representatives, and auxilians.

Two-thirds of the respondents surveyed the hospital staff to determine their interest in or opposition to a health promotion services survey. The methods most often used, in order of frequency of response, were:
- Personal interviews
- Group meetings
- Written questionnaires

The title of the departments most frequently identified as responsible for programs was listed in order of frequency of response:
- Health education and training
- Community health
- Health promotion
- Administration

- Occupational health
- Planning and development

Several individual hospitals also indicated that the following departments are responsible for developing health promotion programs: marketing, cardiac rehabilitation, family practice, personnel, ambulatory care, and outreach services.

Staffing

Eighty percent of the respondents reported that they used existing staff to conduct health promotion programs for business and industry.

If the hospital did hire new staff, the positions they were most likely to add, in order of frequency of response, were:

- Manager of health education
- Exercise physiologist or fitness coordinator
- Physicians
- Consultant
- Clerical staff
- Marketing staff

When asked how many full-time staff provide health promotion services, the following numbers were most frequently mentioned:

- 5 staff persons
- 2 persons
- 5 or more persons
- 3 persons
- 4 persons
- 1 person

In-House Employee Programs

Eighty percent of the respondents indicated that they offered health promotion programs to their own employees before marketing these programs to businesses.

Facilities

Thirty percent of the respondents indicated that either they had built a new facility or they had renovated existing space in order to conduct programs:

- Eighteen hospitals stated they had renovated existing space in such diverse facilities as a warehouse, doctor's office, nursing residence, vacant house, or a kiosk in a shopping mall.
- Four hospitals indicated they had constructed new facilities—either fitness centers or clinical offices.
- Three hospitals leased new space to conduct programs.

Program Sales

When asked how much time had elapsed between initial program development and their first sales call, the period of time mentioned, according to frequency of response, was:

- 1 year
- 6 months
- 1-2 months

When asked how much time had elapsed between the first sales call and actual program sale, the time period mentioned, according to frequency of response, was:

- Within the same month
- 3-4 months
- 1-2 months
- Within 6 months

Funding and Revenue

The most common source of program start-up funding, in order of frequency of response, was:

- Direct hospital operating funds
- Donations
- Grants

The amount of start-up money allocated for program development, in order of frequency of response, was:

- $25,000—$50,000
- $50,000—$100,000
- $100,000—$150,000
- $150,000 or more

Separate Corporate Structure

Seven hospitals reported that they had set up a separate corporate structure for health promotion programs. Twenty-one additional hospitals indicated that they intend to do so in the future.

Fees and Expenses

Respondents reported the following program fees:

- Employee assistance program charges ranged from $3.50 to $22.00 per capita per year.
- Physical examinations and screening charges were $25 and up.
- Life-style educational program fees ranged from $10 to $100 per participant per course or a total program charge of $100 to $675 to a business to conduct a class.

Ninety percent of the respondents indicated that they expected the programs to break even. Eighty percent expected the programs to make a profit. The majority of respondents indicated they expected this to happen in 3 to 5 years.

Marketing to Clients

Approximately one-half of the respondents indicated that they presently had 10 or fewer business clients. The remaining hospitals were providing programs to an average of 25 or more businesses.

The average size of businesses that the hospitals are marketing services to are, in order of frequency of response:

- 100-500 employees (73 percent)
- Fewer than 100 employees (54 percent)
- 500 or more employees (43 percent)

The types of program support provided by the employer that were most frequently mentioned by the hospital are, in order of frequency of response:

- Scheduling of activities
- Facilities or space
- Promotion
- Employee input
- Clerical staff

In evaluating the effectiveness of the health promotion programs, the criteria most frequently used by hospitals are, in order of frequency of response:

- Employee feedback
- Employee participation
- Decreased absenteeism
- Reduced health insurance costs
- Reduced workers' compensation claims

The methods most frequently used to promote health promotion services to business and industry are, in order of frequency of response:

- Individual sales calls
- Promotional mailing
- Group sales meetings
- Advertising

Hospital Consultants

Twenty-eight hospitals indicated that they provide consultation to other hospitals to help them develop health promotion programs. Nineteen of these hospitals charge a fee for these services.

Developmental Problems

The problems most frequently cited by the respondents as inhibiting program development are, in order of frequency of response:

- Inadequate cost-effectiveness data
- Poor local economy resulting in employer cutbacks
- Lack of marketing expertise
- Medical staff opposition
- Inadequate staff to conduct programs
- Inadequate developmental funds
- Lack of employer interest
- Lack of available space at the hospital or work site to conduct programs
- Lack of interest from hospital staff

Reasons for Not Marketing Programs to Business and Industry

Respondents who reported that they were not marketing health promotion services to business and industry were asked to identify why the hospital had decided not to develop programs. The reasons most frequently cited by respondents, in order of frequency of response, were:

- Administration was not convinced that the program was viable.
- Hospital would not invest necessary funds.
- Other businesses were already offering services.
- There was a lack of interest from local business and industry.

Other frequently mentioned responses indicating why the hospital was not presently marketing services to industry were:

- The hospital's current focus was on developing in-house programs for the hospital's employees before marketing programs to businesses.
- The hospital's involvement in other issues, such as building expansion, inpatient services, and corporate restructuring, took precedence over health promotion.
- Physicians were expressing resistance to program development.
- There was a lack of personnel to develop and staff programs.

Appendix B

Corporate Structures For Health Promotion Activities

By Robert H. Rosenfield, Esq., attorney at law,
Memel, Jacobs, Pierno & Gersh, Los Angeles

Increased net revenues are essential to *maintain* our existing hospital system in this age of cost containment. Hospitals must maintain the quality of care as labor and other costs increase, and they must continue to replace fixed assets.

Further, increases in net revenues are needed to *improve* the existing system. Growing, aging communities present new needs. Access to care and quality of care must be improved, and costly technological advancements must be financed.

Unfortunately, recent and dramatic changes in government policies are *reducing* net revenues. This situation will lead to a deterioration of existing facilities and service unless something is done. In addition, increasingly burdensome and restrictive regulation is reducing freedom of action for health care facilities.

Health promotion programs can be effective revenue producers and provide a valuable community service as well. But health care institutions beginning new health promotion programs may also want to consider new legal structures.

Existing Legal Structures

Legal structures should effectively help organizations accomplish their goals. When there have been significant changes in the regulatory or operating environment for organizations, changes in legal structures are usually appropriate. In the investor-owned sector of our economy, frequent change in legal structure has been quite common. On the not-for-profit side, however, particularly in the hospital industry, few organizations have modified the legal structures that emerged during the 1930s and 1940s, despite significant changes in the regulatory and operating environments in which they exist.

Historically, not-for-profit organizations, especially hospitals, have not been greatly concerned with legal structure. There was little need for them to be. Government regulators have shown only benign interest in health care for many years. Only recently has the industry had to live with a pattern of regulation that is both complex and hostile.

One consequence of this dramatic change is that far greater care is called for in planning new activities, especially those that are intended to produce new revenues. Unless this care is taken, new activities may result in unnecessary certificate-of-need (CON) applications, increased taxation, reduced reimbursement, reduced hospital rates, and conceivably all four, rather than increased economic strength. The key to planning strategies for generating new revenues and protecting existing assets is the proper use of legal structures.

Existing Free-Standing Facility

A typical legal structure for hospitals is shown in figure 1. Organized as single not-for-profit organizations, they are exempt from federal and state income taxation (§501(c)(3); §23701d, *California Revenue & Taxation Code*). But as

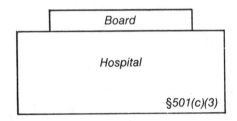

Figure 1. Typical legal structure—existing free-standing facility

single corporations, hospitals are affected by a combination of regulatory programs that could undermine the viability of existing and proposed health promotion activities. For example, hospitals may become vulnerable in the areas of reimbursement, rate setting, taxes, and certificate of need.

Reimbursement

The following need to be considered when discussing reimbursement:

- *Overhead allocations.* Medicare will not reimburse any of the direct costs associated with health promotion activities. In addition, Medicare rules call for a portion of the hospital's overhead (general and administrative expense) to be allocated to such activities. Our experience is that these overhead allocations have been disproportionately large and operate as a penalty on the hospital for engaging in them.
- *Investment income offsets.* Medicare offsets investment income generated from earnings against interest expense.
- *Treatment of gifts and grants.* Gifts that are deemed restricted to operations of a particular department are offset against the costs of that department for the year in which the gift is received. Charitable gifts intended to support health promotion programs might be treated by Medicare as restricted to a reimbursable area, unless care is used.

Rate Setting

Problems similar to those created under reimbursement arise under state rate-setting regulations. If revenue generated by health promotion activities is taken into account by a rate-setting agency, the result could be a failure to obtain a desired hospital rate increase. However, the problems are more serious here because they affect all charges imposed on a health care facility, not just the cost-reimbursed portion of the patient population.

Tax

Recently the Internal Revenue Service shifted more than 150 agents out of employee-benefit-plan work and into the exempt-organization area. The impact of this shift is being felt in California. The California Hospital Association reports that more than 50 times as many audit inquiry letters were received in 1979 as in 1978. The IRS has also instituted a large-case program calling for regular audits of hospitals with more than $10 million in assets. This increase in manpower and focus necessitates greater care in order to avoid or minimize unrelated business income tax that may be imposed on health promotion revenue.

Certificate of Need

Most states now have laws that require hospitals to obtain a CON for any capital expenditure "by" a health facility. This is arguably true even though the capital expenditure has nothing at all to do with direct patient care, for example, expenditures for an educational or health promotional facility.

Controlled Foundations

Hospitals with *controlled* foundations operate as two not-for-profit corporations (figure 2). Both are exempt from federal and state income taxation (§501(c)(3); (§23701d, *California Revenue & Taxation Code*). The hospital

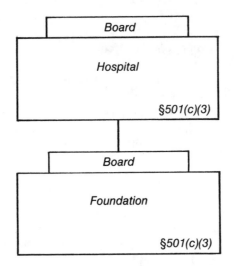

Figure 2. Typical legal structure—existing hospitals with controlled foundations

controls the foundation through the power to appoint and remove board members, and the foundation qualifies as a public charity pursuant to §509(a)(3): that is, support organization. Limitations and vulnerabilities for health promotion programs are in the areas of CON and reimbursement.

Certificate of Need

Because a controlled foundation is not a "health facility," it may be able to make some capital expenditures without a CON. However, in view of limited resources and hospital control, this is not a strong position.

Reimbursement

Accounting rules affecting controlled foundations have been confused. The following points must be considered:

The old *Hospital Audit Guide* called for combined financial reporting for related organizations if "significant resources or operations of a hospital are handled by such organization . . . and they . . . are under control of (or common control with)" the hospital.

There was little consistency of accounting treatment under the former guides. According to AICPA, Accounting Standards Division, *Reporting Practices Concerning Certain Hospital Related Organizations,* Statement of Position 81-2 (August 1, 1981), "the guide does not give sufficient guidance about or explanation of what constitutes 'control' or 'hospital resources.' As a consequence, a variety of reporting practices are being followed and the financial statements of some related organizations are combined with those of hospitals, while the financial statements of other organizations in similar circumstances are not. The related facts and circumstances are sometimes disclosed and sometimes not disclosed."

Statement 81-2, which superseded the old *Hospital Audit Guide* on the issue of combined financial reporting, refers to Accounting Research Bulletin No. 51, *Consolidated Financial Statements,* for guidance on whether the financial statements of related organizations should be consolidated or combined.

Questions still exist under this new test. Many accountants believe that the financial statements of a related not-for-profit organization would have to be consolidated or combined with the financial statement of a not-for-profit hospital that controls any such related not-for-profit organization. Consolidation for financial reporting purposes may lead to consolidation for regulatory purposes as well. Others, however, believe that combined or consolidated financial statements would not be required because there is no ownership of the related organization as required under Accounting Research Bulletin No. 51.

Regardless of which interpretation is followed, Statement 81-2 clearly requires elaborate footnote disclosure on the financial statements of not-for-profit hospitals or other not-for-profit organizations that are *related* under the tests set forth in Statement 81-2. A separate organization is considered to be related to a hospital if: "(i) the hospital controls the separate organization through contracts or other legal documents that provide to the hospital the authority to direct the separate organization's activities, management, and policies, or (ii) the hospital is for all practical purposes the sole beneficiary of an organization." Such footnoting will leave an "audit trail," which could cause third-party organizations to seek to affect, by rules, regulations, and practices, the assets of the related organization.

Medicare regulations now provide for application of generally accepted accounting principles. However, comparable attitudes may develop in the certificate-of-need area or among rate-setting agencies if an attempt is made to use controlled foundations as a base from which to conduct new activities that would be regulated if done directly by the hospital.

Because the foundation is controlled by the hospital, any new programs calling for a sale of services by the foundation to the hospital will be covered by the related organization principle. The hospital will be reimbursed only for the costs to the foundation of providing such services.

The controlled foundation has existed for many years in the hospital industry. However, it is doubtful it will provide a preferable corporate structure for conducting health promotion activities. Despite the provisions of Statement 81-2 and A.R.B. 51, the threat that the corporate entities will be ignored for regulatory purposes is so great that we would encourage consideration of other alternatives.

New Legal Structures

Two new legal structures are the independent foundation and the parent corporation.

The Independent Foundation

The independent foundation is organized as shown in figure 3 and falls under not-for-profit corporation law. It is exempt from federal income tax.

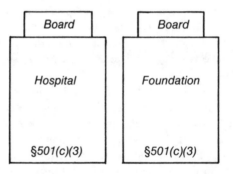

Figure 3. New legal structure—independent foundation

It is essential that the independent foundation avoid "private-foundation" status under the Internal Revenue Code. Otherwise, donors will be denied a full charitable deduction on contributions, and organizations will be subject to severe penalty taxes and other irritations.

Traditionally, hospital foundations have avoided private-foundation status by way of §509(a)(3) of the Internal Revenue Code. However, because §509(a)(3) requires that the foundation be "operated, supervised, or controlled by or in connection with the hospital," going this route would jeopardize separate regulatory and accounting treatment.

The alternative to §509(a)(3) is §509(a)(1), which incorporates by reference the "publicly supported" organization tests described in §170(b)(1)(a)(vi). Whether or not an organization can meet the tests set forth in that section depends on the nature of its activities and the amount of support it can obtain from the general public. Care must be taken in this area.

If the independence of a foundation is to be recognized for regulatory purposes, the hospital cannot be in a position to control its affairs. Note, however, that the concept of control varies considerably under different regulatory programs. Compare, for example, the detailed treatment given this subject by the accounting profession in Statement 81-2 (referred to earlier) with the complete absence of any discussion of related organization concepts in CON laws. Other, and different, tests can be found in the Internal Revenue Code, Medicare regulations, and general corporate concepts. Clearly, it is critical to structure an independent foundation with a view to accomplish an objective under particular governmental programs rather than in the abstract. Only with particular tests in mind should a structure be developed.

Most controlled hospital foundations have clauses in their articles of incorporation that require the hospital to receive all the funds raised by the foundation. While such clauses, standing alone, might not destroy the foundation's independence, they are dangerous. Preferably, purposes clauses should limit the foundation to supporting health care facilities within a certain geographical area. Ideally, the foundation should be given sufficient flexibility to make grants to a variety of organizations other than the hospital. A consistent pattern of giving to other organizations would provide helpful evidence of independence should the status of the foundation be challenged.

It is possible to obtain additional influence over the affairs of a foundation by contract. If real estate is to be transferred to an independent foundation, restrictions can be placed in the terms of any ground lease, deed, or mortgage that is used in connection with the transfer. However, these restrictions must not be so burdensome as to destroy the foundation's independence for regulatory purposes. The hospital can also obtain pledges from the foundation in order to be certain that it will get funds from the foundation when it needs them. Properly drafted, these pledges should be enforceable at law, and this, in turn, will satisfy lenders when a project is adequately capitalized.

Depending on the terms of the hospital's indenture or loan documents, it may be technically impossible to transfer significant assets to the independent foundation. For example, if the hospital already has an education building, consideration might be given to transferring it to the new, independent foundation. This may eliminate some of the reimbursement, rate-setting, and certificates-of-need problems. However, we generally do not recommend significant asset transfers to independent foundations. The price, in terms of control, is generally too great to justify the benefits.

Limiting the number of hospital affiliated directors is easily the most important way to determine whether or not the foundation is controlled by the hospital. Certainly the hospital should not have an ability to appoint a majority of the board. Many alternative approaches are possible:

- Requiring the foundation board to select a certain number of directors from the hospital board.
- Limiting the number of hospital directors to a specified percentage of the foundation's board (for example, 10 percent or 33 percent).
- Using former board members to some extent.
- Using a clause in the articles of incorporation that would provide that at no time shall the board have more than a specified percentage of its membership made up of directors who are affiliated with any single hospital or health facility. *Affiliated* is defined in the bylaws to mean an officer, director, employee, agent, or member of the medical staff. If the percentage limitation is violated (as a result of vacancies) the president of the organization is obligated to suspend those directors who are affiliated until the percentage limitation is complied with.

Potential problems include diverging objectives and even conflict if the foundation is controlled by the hospital and dependent on the hospital even if organized as an independent form.

The Parent Corporation

Use of parent-type organizations (see figure 4, opposite) is widespread in other highly regulated industries, especially banking and utilities. The key concept used is that, generally speaking, assets and revenues of the parent are not reflected on the financial statements of its subsidiaries. This raises the possibility that the parent can engage in many activities that would be regulated if conducted directly by a hospital subsidiary.

The parent organization is organized under not-for-profit corporation law. Parents are the sole members of the existing hospital corporation, which gives them the power to appoint and remove board members of the subsidiary at will. When the existing hospital corporation has numerous public members, difficulties may arise. Consider transferring memberships in the hospital subsidiary to memberships in the new parent. Properly understood, this should eliminate opposition.

Purposes clauses are the most important provisions in the articles of incorporation. They define the terms of the charitable trust (holding of assets for the general public) and may lock the parent into particular activities. Making the parent's purposes virtually identical to those of the hospital should

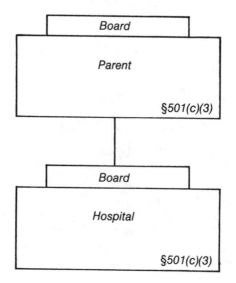

Figure 4. New legal structure—parent corporation

eliminate the charitable trust problem, because the transferred assets will still be subject to the same trust. However, broader purposes will permit greater flexibility in terms of what activities the parent will want to undertake in the future.

Parent corporations should apply for federal and state income-tax exemptions.

A problem under §170(b)(1)(a)(vi) is that if the parent board is to be identical to the subsidiary's board, the new structure will not be able to bring in new faces to be responsible for fund raising. Some organizations have successfully used advisory boards to perform this function.

If the parent's activities generate the wrong kind of income, the parent may be unable to meet either of the public support tests. If a foundation exists or is planned, a concerted fund-raising effort by the parent would be counterproductive. But it may be possible to use hospital or foundation grants to the parent to meet the public support test.

Many hospitals have assets that might well be transferred to a parent. Some of these are operating surpluses, endowment assets, medical office buildings, parking lots, and education and research facilities. Revenue from these activities can be used to support startup costs of health promotion programs. However, there are many legal questions that must be resolved before such action can be taken:

- Will the hospital be giving up meaningful opportunities to bury costs by transferring health promotion activities to the parent?
- Revenues of the parent's health promotion activities might be deemed to reduce the parent's costs. This could be a particular concern if the parent functions as a home office. Will this be a problem?
- Is there an effect on tax exemption or the public foundation status?
- Do you want a separate board of directors?

Review and Modification of Corporate Structure

A number of steps should be taken before work begins on a detailed analysis. In our experience, these steps can be very important:

- *Educate your board.* Many hospital trustees are prominent in their communities and devoted to the hospital and its future, but we have met few who have a clear picture of the readily changing regulatory environment in which hospitals must function. In view of the complexity of this pattern, it is not surprising. However, it is important that the trustees have a clear idea of what is happening today if they are going to be receptive to major changes in the corporate structure. Present each board member with written materials on the subject of corporate restructuring and conduct an educational session for the board. These sessions can last from 1½ hours (on the short side) to full-day retreats. Properly handled, these programs will significantly increase trustee understanding and involvement with a corporate restructuring project.
- *Assemble a team of advisers.* If the board wants to explore corporate restructuring, its next step should be to assemble a team of experienced professionals. The team should consist of qualified legal and accounting professionals who are familiar with hospital regulations and reporting in general and the issues relating to corporate restructuring in particular.
- *Form a steering committee.* Frequent communication with the board is essential to successful corporate restructuring. Many boards will prefer this function be undertaken by a committee. Define the committee's role and determine who will serve.
- *Analyze the existing structure.* Once the team is assembled, the first step will be to review all relevant documentation concerning the hospital's existing structure from a regulatory and reporting standpoint. Among others, review the hospital's long-range plan; Medicare and Medicaid cost reports; forms 990 and 990-T (if any); financial statements, articles of incorporation, and bylaws; all bond indentures, mortgages, and deeds of trust; and preliminary title reports or title insurance policies showing all real estate owned and the location of principal buildings.
- *Focus the study.* When the document review and analysis has been

completed, meet with the board or committee to discuss findings and to focus on those areas the board is most interested in incorporating into the restructuring study. This is an important stage. Frequently, hospitals have a lengthy list of ideas, all of which could be incorporated into the study. However, if too many ideas are factored into the analysis, it will raise the project cost significantly and add to its complexity. It is far better to focus the study on existing problems and opportunities. Most structures can be easily modified in the future to accommodate changes and new developments.

Proposal Development

The following steps are involved in developing proposals for corporate restructuring:

- *Interviews.* Interviews of selected administration and board personnel should be a part of the corporate restructuring process. The number and duration of these interviews can be tailored to the tastes of particular organizations. They can be conducted prior to focusing the study, if desired, but will be lengthier because a wider variety of subjects will have to be covered. We prefer conducting the interviews after the board has indicated which areas should be covered by the study. Confidential interviews can then reveal the true feelings of key individuals and help to ensure that recommended proposals will be adopted.
- *Legal research and analysis.* A thorough review must be made of the legal issues presented by a particular project. Hospitals are subject to audit by many agencies. Any proposed change in legal structure or location of assets must be analyzed to assure the board that the new structure will be worthwhile from the standpoint of cost-benefit analysis.
- *Financial analysis.* New structures and activities must be analyzed from a financial perspective. New construction must have adequate cash flow to be completed and to fund operating deficits in the early years, and new corporate structures must produce new reporting relationships if they are to be effective from a reimbursement standpoint. Pro forma cost reports and tax returns should be prepared so the board will understand what the dollar consequences of various legal structures are likely to be.
- *Preliminary proposals.* Once the interviews and legal and financial analyses have been completed, the professionals, working closely with administration, will develop preliminary proposals concerning legal structure and assets transfers. These preliminary proposals will be presented to the board (or committee) for their consideration.
- *Preparing draft study.* Once the preliminary proposals have been developed and approved, the professionals should formalize the recommendations and document their findings. This document will set forth

in full the legal and financial analysis that underlie the recommendations.

- *Presentation and discussion.* When a draft study has been completed, excerpts should be circulated among members of the board (or committee). Two weeks or so after the excerpts have been circulated, a meeting should be held during which the professionals and administration formally present the results of the study. The length of the discussion process and the persons involved will necessarily vary from institution to institution.
- *Implementation.* When a new structure has been approved, a variety of steps need to be taken for implementation. New corporate entities need be created. New articles of incorporation and bylaws must be prepared, boards named, and officers appointed. Not-for-profit corporations that desire tax exemption must apply for determination letters; substantial asset transfers will necessitate rulings from the national office of the IRS. Documents of transfer must be drawn up, and where necessary, approvals must be obtained from lenders, regulators, and others.

In addition to these outlined steps, a number of operating considerations, such as number of staff, employee benefits, accounting systems and reporting formats, office space, and sources of initial financing, must be taken into consideration.

Any new legal structure will require a process of education and change of habits for most persons, whether they be board members or employees. It is important that new corporate structures be respected by the organization if they are going to be respected by third parties.

Become sensitive to new developments that may call for further modification to the legal structure. Corporate restructuring should be considered a continuing process. If a hospital contemplates an acquisition, the creation of a new nonreimbursable cost center, or the development of a piece of real estate, consideration should be given to the legal form in which that activity should be conducted.

Watch for regulatory changes. Dramatic changes in regulatory and reporting programs must be anticipated in the next five years. Try to ensure that you stay aware of these changes and of any implications they may have for your legal structure. Particular arrangements may be adversely affected by regulatory changes in the future and may call for further modifications of corporate structure in order to prevent adverse consequences.

Bibliography

The bibliography is a basic set of readings on the subject of health promotion in the work place and is not intended to be all-inclusive. Articles and books were chosen according to the following minimum criteria:

- That studies have been validated in the work setting or at least could be generalized to the work place.
- That studies or reviews of studies have considered a reasonable evaluation framework for determining the effectiveness of prevention programs.
- That books or articles purporting to discuss the cost-benefit or cost-effectiveness of prevention programs do indeed consider both sides of the equation of a cost-benefit analysis, including the social costs, if possible.
- That resource materials on planning and developing employee health programs take into account results from a wide variety of business and governmental experiences and avoid reinventing the wheel.
- That authors have raised critical problems and issues affecting policy questions that all parties involved with employee health programs must face.
- That the resources provide a conceptual framework or model for development of disease prevention programs.

Background Studies

The General Mills American Family Report 1978-1979: Family Health in an Era of Stress. Minneapolis: General Mills, Inc., 1979.

In a national study conducted by Yankelovich, Skelly and White. Inc.. a probability sample of 1,254 families were surveyed on the following topics: (1) the impact of inflation on family health attitudes and concerns, (2) barriers to good health, (3) personal values and their impact on health attitudes and behavior, (4) preventive versus crisis health care, (5) physical fitness, (6) health parenting, (8) mental illness, (9) health issues, and (10) levels of information about health practices. A large panel of experts was part of an initial phase that helped to generate hypotheses worth testing. Results were reported mainly for the principal adult respondents (spouses and teenagers were also interviewed), because they comprised a majority of interviewees.

Key findings suggest that families tend to have great faith in physicians to solve their health problems when they occur but appear reluctant to have physical checkups as a means for prevention and tend to delay in seeking medical care not considered necessary. They also reported that manifestations of emotional and mental health problems are the result of personal weakness and expressed a desire to handle such problems without seeking professional help. According to the researchers, families think there will be a cure for cancer in their lifetime and engage in denial about the prospect of catastrophic illness, or even mental illness, happening to them, although at least one-fourth of the adult population smoked and around two-thirds did not exercise regularly. There was evidence of an awareness of major risk factors for chronic diseases and what to do about them but lack of knowledge on how to follow through on needed behavioral changes.

Though this study was not conducted in the work place, it is one of the few national health information, utilization, and behavior studies commissioned by a large industrial concern. Making interpretations from this and applying them in the work place should be done cautiously as the study design and analysis did not provide for generalizability of results in selected populations.

The study is available from General Mills, Inc., 9200 Wayzata Boulevard, Minneapolis, MN 55440.

Goldbeck, Willis, and Kiefhaber, Anne. Wellness: the new employee benefit. *Group Practice Journal.* 30:20-21, Mar. 1981.

The authors of this paper review program examples and trends seen in the business sector to help keep health care costs down. The programs most identified with the occupational wellness movement are those that provide educational facilities or incentives for health enhancement and life-style changes.

Pearson, Clarence E. *Education for Health in the Workplace.* New York City: Metropolitan Life Insurance Company, 1979.

In this paper Pearson presents an international perspective through the description of data obtained from a survey of large multinational corporations with headquarters located in North America and Europe. The survey was commissioned by the International Health Resource Consortium Committee on Health Education/Information Exchange Systems. The 83 responding plants were located in Africa, Asia, the Middle East, the Americas, and Europe; a majority employed 500 or more workers.

The data relate the type of health services and promotional programs conducted, the chief techniques used, the types of personnel employed to design and implement health education programs, and the success rate for screening programs in the industrial setting. There appears to be strong interest among respondents about acquiring information on health education programs and in learning how to establish health promotion programs.

Included in the paper is a valuable set of guidelines for program development and evaluation techniques to produce indicators of short-term success in controlling hospital and medical expenses for long-term illness. It is available from Metropolitan Life Insurance Company, One Madison Avenue, New York, NY 10010 (212/578-6441).

Proceedings of the National Conference on Health Promotion Programs in Occupational Settings. Washington, DC: Government Printing Office, 1979.

The proceedings offer an excellent summary of a set of background papers that delve into the state of the art of eight different components of health promotion referred to in the proceedings as risk reduction components. Risk reduction and assessment of individual mortality and morbidity for cardiovascular disease, cancer, and stroke that could be linked with the risk reduction programs constitute the major definition of a health promotion program at the work site, according to the conference planners.

The eight different components of health promotion included smoking control, weight control, nutrition and dietary practices, hypertension control, exercise and fitness, drug and alcohol abuse control, stress management, and accidents and self-protection against work-place hazards. Other issues addressed in the conference involved questions related to the appropriateness of program design and administration, the purposes and elements of information systems, union and management relations, physician views of occupational medicine, the types and elements of an evaluation plan, the cost-effectiveness of a health promotion program, and the measurements used in making such analyses. Individual papers will be annotated elsewhere under specific headings.

A Report on Lifestyle/Personal Health Care in Different Occupations. Kansas City, MO: Academy of Family Physicians, 1979.

The study, conducted by a private search firm, surveyed the attitudes and practices of a randomly selected sample of six occupational groups who are members of six professional, union, and fraternal organizations cutting across hundreds of work sites in the United States. The six occupational groups included business executives, family physicians, farmers, garment workers, secretaries, and teachers. Nearly 10,000 persons responded to questions on work, home, stress, life-styles, medical problems, access to health care, and the integration of health, or the means by which respondents cope with stress and patterns of health care they pursue.

Results for each domain varied by occupation, and researchers interpreted this as an indication of a lack of a consistent, integrated approach toward healthy living. Sources of stress on the job provoked reactions such as overeating, abuse of alcohol, tobacco, and so forth, just as did problems associated with health, home, and sex life. Thus, the researchers concluded that there is a need for greater understanding of the connections between work, stress, and health which might increase the integration of healthier life-styles in all aspects of individuals' lives.

Implications of the findings for the practitioner include taking a more comprehensive approach in the development, implementation, and evaluation of life-style intervention in the work place in addition to instituting isolated exercise and fitness, nutritional, and other categorical self-help and stress programs. The conclusion to be reached is that there is a need to recognize that a more fundamental issue is at stake. Life-style change may not be readily sustained over time through a piecemeal approach to treating symptoms instead of underlying problems associated with the work place. Their findings were based on correlation analysis only, and it is not clear whether generalizations about all workers and all work sites can be made from these findings. The study is available from Academy of Family Physicians, 1740 West 42nd Street, Kansas City, MO 64114.

Survey of Industry Sponsored Health Promotion, Prevention, and Education Programs. Washington, DC: Washington Business Group on Health, 1978.

Data on 13 different programs was obtained from only 50 of 160 companies who are members of the Washington Business Group on Health. It was stressed that most health promotion programs in occupational settings were begun after 1970, with over half begun since 1975. Little data on effectiveness and/or cost-benefit analysis was used as a basis for program initiation. Much of the survey data was deemed to be soft data because of incomplete or nonexistent answers to survey questions. Ranking of problems, evaluation criteria, and reasons for program initiation were determined. Major methods of communication, sources of program initiation, availability to employees, utilization patterns, frequency of services provided, and insurance coverage were tabulated. Data on costs were not available. Few, if any, conclusions can be drawn from this purely descriptive study because of its methodological flaws. However, this interim report could give insight to practitioners into the milieu in which health promotion programs are conducted in some work settings. The study is available from Washington Business Group on Health, 605 Pennsylvania Avenue, S.E., Washington, DC 20003 (202/547-6700).

Weinberg, Andrew, and others. *Health Promotion in the Community: A Guide to Working with Employers.* Washington, DC: Washington Business Group on Health, 1980.

The Washington Business Group on Health is a membership organization of 200 leading corporations concerned with employee well-being, responsible cost management, and sound health policy. More than 50,000,000 employees, retirees, and their dependents receive health and medical benefits from these employers. Starting in 1977, health promotion and mental wellness have been high-priority issues on which the staff has worked at the national and local levels with WBGH member companies. This paper is designed to give the reader a general understanding of the current status of health promotion programs in industry. It is available from Washington Business Group on Health, 605 Pennsylvania Avenue, S.E., Washington, DC 20003 (202/547-6700).

Planning and Developing Programs

Berry, Charles A. *Good Health for Employees and Reduced Health Care Costs for Industry.* Washington, DC: Health Insurance Association of America, 1981.

This publication was developed to provide businesses with good, basic information on the importance of developing work-site health promotion programs to help identify and reduce employee health risks. The publication describes health promotion programs being conducted by businesses throughout the country, cites examples of estimated cost savings by individual businesses, and outlines initial planning steps and strategies to help industry develop programs for their employees. It is available from Health Insurance Association of America, 1850 K Street, N.W., Washington, DC 20006 (202/862-4029).

Cooper, Philip D., and others, editors. *Marketing and Preventive Health Care: Interdisciplinary and Interorganizational Perspectives.* Chicago: American Marketing Association, 1978.

The emphasis throughout this publication is to avoid viewing the marketing of preventive care as the selling of health care services to consumers who already want such a product and to assume a standard of success other than 100 percent, which is the typical expectation when a new program is instituted in the health care field. The need for well-conceived market research is underscored, and two excellent examples of market research, one applied to family planning and the other to consumer attitudes and social influences associated with health care services, is carefully presented.

Appropriate definitions of marketing are made. An apparent problem is that health care practitioners have equated selling and slick advertising approaches with marketing. They are either suspicious of marketing techniques or have completely misapplied marketing techniques and so have compromised their own efforts in health promotion.

Other cautionary concerns were raised. Two of these are the need to consider the initial costs of developing a sound marketing approach toward prevention because major funds are usually required in the beginning for quality research, and tangible results are not always reached in a short time frame because prevention is not always a tangible commodity. Because of this, standards for success must be measured in more specific terms.

Lazes, Peter M., editor. *The Handbook of Health Education.* Germantown, MD: Aspen Systems, 1979.

This book provides a tool for understanding and developing health education programs in several settings. Of special note are background chapters on job safety and health and health education in health maintenance organizations for their application to the business or industrial setting. In the sections on self-care and media for community health promotion, results of studies on the effectiveness of projects and programs are described in terms of short-term and intermediate outcomes. The section on exercise and fitness includes methods for instituting new programs, and the nutrition section presents new dietary goals and guidelines in reference to maintaining health and reducing obesity. These chapters and the extensive resource list of books, periodicals, and groups in the appendix will aid those wishing to tailor an employee health program to the needs of the participants in practical and realistic terms.

A Practical Guide for Employee Health Promotion Programs. Madison, WI: Health Planning Council, Feb. 1979.

This guide defines components of an employee health promotion program and describes the types of services that should be included. It also begins from the assumption that no program can be instituted without the identification of individual health risks and the modification of those risks. An entire section is devoted to a summary of the health and cost benefits of various employee health programs that were studied in both the public and private sector. The guide also provides a handy format for gathering base-line information on health-related costs and outlines the how-to of developing an administratively sound program. It also summarizes several employee health programs across the country and includes a major section on resource persons and organizations. It is available from Health Planning Council, 310 Price Place, Suite 206, Madison, WI 53705.

Sehnert, Keith W., and Tillotson, John K. *A National Health Care Strategy: How Business Can Promote Good Health for Employees and Their Families.* Washington, DC: The National Chamber Foundation, 1978.

The audience for this booklet is primarily business executives who would be investigating the need for a health promotion program for their respective firms and the potential savings in insurance benefits and disability time that might be accrued from instituting such a program. Such information is also useful to the practitioner interested in working with businessmen in instituting new programs. Written and printed in a highly readable style, the report gives a short summary of why business would benefit from an involvement in health promotion, including findings from key studies in prevention. Fourteen health promotion programs (or components of health promotion programs) are considered in a format that includes a short statement of the problem, potential solutions or approaches, suggestions for program evaluation, examples of ongoing programs in business, and resources for information. A final chapter outlines a step-by-step action plan with scorecards provided for gathering base-line data for pilot projects. The appendixes report on selected case studies of corporate health promotion programs and provide some key references and resources. It is available from the National Chamber Foundation, 1615 H Street, N.W., Washington, DC 20062 (202/659-6188).

Thomas, Jane. *Promoting Health in the Worksetting.* Madison, WI: Institute for Health Planning, 1981.

This paper discusses the cost-savings potential of work-site health promotion programs, the components and keys to a successful work-site program, and ways in which the health planning agency can provide assistance to community businesses in establishing or expanding these programs. The paper also includes a section on selected organizational resources for work-site health promotion programs. It is available from the Institute for Health Planning, 702 North Blackhawk Avenue, Madison, WI 53705 (608/233-9791).

Costs and Benefits

Cardiovascular Primer for the Workplace. Bethesda, MD: Office of Prevention, Education, and Control, National Institutes of Health, Jan. 1981. (NIH publication no. 81-2210)

This booklet was developed by the Office of Prevention, Education, and Control of the National Heart, Lung, and Blood Institute as a tool to make corporate managers aware of the impact of cardiovascular disease on employee health. In addition to factual information about the prevalence of hypertension and other cardiovascular-related illnesses, it provides employers with such practical information as factors to consider in beginning a prevention program and possible resources that can be tapped to help get a program off the ground. It also contains an excellent section entitled "Economics, Cardiovascular Disease and Workers," which includes statistics on the costs of cardiovascular-disease-related medical care to the employer. It is available from Coordinator for Workplace Activities, Health Education Branch, Office of Prevention, Education, and Control, National Heart, Lung, and Blood Institute, Building 31, Room 4A18, Bethesda, MD 20205.

Fielding, Jonathan E. Evaluation of worksite health promotion programs. In: *Institute of Medicine Conference Summary: Evaluating Health Promotion in the Workplace.* Washington, DC: Institute of Medicine, Jan. 1981.

In this extensive paper, Fielding indicates that evaluation of work-site health promotion programs is at a very early stage of development. The heterogeneous nature of programs subsumed under the rubric of health promotion makes it difficult to generalize about the current state of evaluation efforts. However, based on the Center for Health Enhancement's experience in working with several private businesses and not-for-profit organizations, a number of steps and related problems are generic to many efforts at evaluation of work-site health promotion programs. The paper identifies some of the limitations common to many evaluation designs and suggests methodological improvements. Better evaluation can reveal hidden costs and benefits and can lead to refinement of programmatic approaches.

_____. Health and industrial relations. In: *Health Care and Industrial Relations: Costs, Conflicts and Controversy.* Los Angeles: Institute of Industrial Relations, University of California—Los Angeles, 1980.

Fielding's overview touches lightly on several of the major industrial health issues, each of which is an appropriate subject for a lengthy paper. What emerges is a picture of the extent and pace of fundamental changes that are occurring in the industrial health area. New and changing programs are altering both labor and management perceptions of their responsibilities and opportunities for both improved health and improved health care delivery systems. Many other developed nations have more stable arrangements for financing of health care and more clearly delineated responsibilities for labor, management, private medicine, and government. Continued experimentation can benefit both labor and management if changes are evaluated qualitatively and quantitatively and if better levels of health care rather than the fullest possible range of health benefits are accepted as a primary goal.

_____. Preventive medicine and the bottom line. Unpublished paper, Massachusetts Department of Public Health, Boston, Aug. 1978.

Fielding performed a thorough review of the literature, examining a variety of major cost-savings claims from employers who have instituted preventive programs at the work site. He also presents a rationale for employers instituting preventive programs, refuting the argument that reduction of direct costs for preventive programs becomes deferred costs rather than savings, because employees will eventually become ill and die of a competing illness. Throughout the literature review, many benefits in monetary terms were cited, but only a few practical examples of employer analyses that compared costs with benefits were included, probably because such examples are rare or at least unusual. However, no programs reporting classic cost-benefit or cost-effectiveness studies were described. As a result of the review, the author advocates that six major proved preventive interventions should be incorporated into a firm's internal health promotion programs. They include hypertension screening and follow-up, smoking cessation, exercise, alcoholism control, auto safety, and diet modification.

Follman Jr., Joseph F. *The Economics of Industrial Health: History, Theory, Practice.* New York City: AMACOM, 1978.

This book is a valuable source for the history, theory, and practice (as its title suggests) of health programs conducted in the work place. The relationship of the Occupational Safety and Health Act of 1970 and the historic movement toward preventive health care (that is, inclusion of health education, changing life-styles, physical examinations, screening, and rehabilitation) to the development of industrial programs is thoroughly described by the author. Industrial programs are described in terms of employer, union, and governmental roles, and the classic health status indicators and economic costs mandating the need for such programs. Of special interest are the last three sections on the current state of the art. In these sections, Follman carefully develops the problems of setting up industrial health programs in terms of all of the necessary steps, including the issues of confidentiality of records, insurance coverage, union cooperation, the supervisor's role, costs involved, and the problems of small employers.

The area of employee assistance programs, including counseling and treatment for mental illness, alcoholism, and drug abuse, is highlighted. The role of public and private financing and insurance programs in prevention and rehabilitation is given a balanced treatment. An important section on the cost-effectiveness of preventive medicine and industrial health programs is critically reviewed, providing detailed interpretations of approaches and themes most likely to succeed.

Finally, the appendixes, which include the Occupational Safety and Health

Act of 1970, information about established industrial programs, resource guides, and an annotated bibliography, are must reading in this most comprehensive approach to the subject of economics and promotion of health and the maintenance of wellness in the work place.

Lave, Judith R., and Lester, B. Cost-benefit concepts in health: examination of some prevention efforts. *Preventive Medicine.* 7:414-23, Sept. 1978.

In this important article, the authors lay out the key reasons for evaluating health programs and then present four steps in the evaluation process. They clearly emphasize comparing both beneficial and negative effects, which have to be quantitatively related to the program and then have to be translated into a single metric (usually dollars) comparing inputs and outputs over time.

These steps were applied to preventive measures such as screening for breast cancer. The problems associated with performing this type of research were discussed. The results of a major literature review performed while the authors cochaired a task force on the Economic Impact of Preventive Medicine are discussed. Only a few studies come close to meeting the above criteria: screening for PKU, immunization programs, multiphasic screening at Kaiser, and screening for breast cancer utilizing mammography. However, results from the Kaiser study were ambiguous, and the results for breast cancer screening were differential, depending on age.

The authors conclude that cost-benefit and cost-effectiveness analyses cannot be the sole criterion for decision making because certain economic issues, such as income distribution and the measurement problems, have not been addressed. General health status measures are the key to efficiency, and a call was made for improved health status indicators and better work in research and development using large populations over longer periods.

Schoeffler, Richard, and Paringer, Lynn. A review of the economic evidence on prevention. *Medical Care.* 18:7, May 1980.

This study examines the economic evidence on prevention and health care. A discussion of cost-benefit analysis and cost-effectiveness analysis, their applications to preventive strategies, and the problems inherent in implementing these approaches precedes a review of the empirical evidence.

Prevention strategies are grouped into three categories: life-style changes, public health measures, and screening programs. Life-style changes include altering behavior patterns as they relate to alcohol and drug abuse, smoking, and automobile safety regulations. Included in public health measures are immunizations against communicable diseases, water fluoridation, and food inspection. Screening includes programs for detection of PKU and congenital hypothyroidism in newborn infants, for spina bifida cystica in the unborn fetus, and hypertension.

The paper concludes that many of the preventive health measures examined represent an efficient use of resources. Because only quantifiable changes in health status or costs are included in the benefit-cost and cost-effectiveness analyses, the actual value of prevention strategies may be understated because reductions in pain and suffering usually are omitted.

What do cost-benefit studies say about health education? *Physician's Patient Education Newsletter.* 2:1-2, Oct. 1979.

A short review of four utilization studies was made. In only two of the studies could a cost-benefit ratio be applied: one on the reduction of emergency department utilization by asthmatics and one on a Cold Self-Care Center established in a prepaid ambulatory care setting. Even results of these studies do not qualify as presenting sufficient evidence to demonstrate that health education is cost-beneficial, because the increased cost of medical care over an individual's lifetime as a result of an increased life expectancy (because of the health education program) must be taken into account when calculating costs.

Because only estimates for such future costs can be used and because most health education programs often increase medical care utilization and therefore increase short-term costs, it is recommended that justification of such programs not be made solely on the basis of a favorable cost-benefit ratio. Long-term measures, such as those expressed in terms of the prevention of illness, improvement of compliance to a therapeutic regimen that leads to a speedier recovery, and the right to being informed of an enhanced quality of life, should be given due consideration in justifying health education programs.

Effective Activities by Category

Alcoholism and Drug Abuse

DuPont, Robert L. The control of alcohol and drug abuse in industry. In: *Proceedings of the National Conference on Health Promotion Programs in Occupational Settings.* Washington, DC: Government Printing Office, 1979.

This background paper extensively reviews 61 recent pieces of literature on the definition, design, and effectiveness of alcohol and drug-abuse control programs that have been instituted in industry to date. The statistics on the extent of the alcohol and drug abuse problem as it relates to job performance and the difficulty of making this type of measurement are explored, along with a description of occupational programs and the ideal goals for such programs outlined in the *Third Special Report to the U.S. Congress on Alcohol and Health.*

DuPont emphasizes the mixed findings of drug-related studies in terms of worker performance as compared with the consistent findings of research on the effect of alcohol on employee behavior. He also summarizes the four dominant models and several interventions used in the most common programs usually labeled as *employee assistance programs.* The impact of various employee assistance programs dealing with alcoholism is reviewed and found to be somewhat effective overall, especially for programs including referral mechanisms. However, assumptions of financial returns on such programs have not been supported because of the lack of sophisticated research designs and unreliable methods of analysis, with the exception of one major military study that employed the use of command directives to mandate participation and make time available for interventions.

The paper also addresses policy issues such as the role of the occupational program consultant as an interface between workers and management rather than as a marketer of a product and the need for variation in programs to suit the special needs of small businesses, women, youth, and multidrug users.

Follmann Jr., J. F. *Alcoholics and Business.* New York City: AMACOM, 1976.

The author outlines what the scope and costs of alcoholism in the work place are, how the alcoholic employee can be identified, what can be done about the problem, what the accomplishments are to date, and where help and guidance can be obtained. The appendixes include information about employer alcoholism programs and list sources of help and guidance.

Jones, K., and Vischi, T. Summary of impact of alcoholism treatment on medical care utilization and cost. In: *National Institute on Alcohol Abuse and Alcoholism Health Insurance Resources Kit,* 1979.

The report contains 12 studies, 9 of which were excerpted from a larger unpublished study by the Alcohol, Drug Abuse and Mental Health Administration, Department of Health, Education, and Welfare in 1979, that included alcoholism, drugs, and mental health. These studies review the impact of alcoholism on medical care utilization and costs. Of the 12 studies, 8 focus on employer-based alcoholism programs and 3 center on alcoholism treatment within a health maintenance organization (HMO) setting.

Eight of the studies found that alcoholism treatment was followed by reductions ranging from 26 percent to 69 percent in medical care utilization. The median reduction for medical care in these studies was 46 percent. Three of these studies calculated the dollar amounts of the reductions and found savings in general health care of 41¢, 45¢, and $1.10 for each dollar spent on the alcoholism programs. Of the three HMO studies, the Group Health Association of America (GHAA) effort was the most significant, because this was the first attempt to systematically examine the feasibility of comprehensive alcoholism services in a prepaid health maintenance organization setting. This study found a 31 percent reduction in utilization of total health services as compared with two years before entering treatment and a 57 percent reduction in family member utilization following the initial treatment of alcoholic family members.

The implication of the studies strongly suggests that treatment for alcohol abuse and alcoholism is frequently followed by a reduction in medical utilization and cost. It should be cautioned, however, that all of the studies do have at least some methodological limitations, such as small study groups, inadequate comparison groups, short-term spans, or only surrogate measures of medical utilization.

Kiefhaber, Anne, and Goldbeck, Willis B. *A WBGH Survey on Employee Mental Wellness Programs*. Washington, DC: Washington Business Group on Health, 1979.

Results of a survey of member company mental health or wellness programs are presented briefly. Membership is confined to 160 of America's largest businesses, which have an economic interest in keeping workers healthy and productive and in saving money on health insurance premiums. Mental illness programs tend to fall under employee assistance efforts in large companies. Data were presented on program initiation, types of services available, utilization, evaluation, and insurance benefits covered or not covered by the various companies.

An overview of many issues is contained in the second section. Included is a definition of a mental wellness program to encompass the following areas: alcohol and drug abuse, psychiatric and psychological problems, life crisis counseling involving financial and legal problems, occupational stress, and insured medical benefits. Ramifications of instituting such a program are given a nice treatment, and two helpful checklists on beginning a model program for mental wellness end the report.

The report is available from: Washington Business Group on Health, 605 Pennsylvania Avenue, S.E., Washington, DC 20003 (202/547-6700).

Schramm, Carl J. Evaluating industrial alcoholism programs. *Journal of Studies on Alcohol*. 41:702-13, 1980.

The author presents a human-capital model for explaining employer decisions regarding initiation or continuation of employee alcoholism treatment programs. An eight-item model for estimating the annual cost of alcoholism to the company is included.

_____. Measuring the return on program costs: evaluation of a multi-employer alcoholism treatment program. *American Journal of Public Health*.

67:50-51, Jan. 1977.

This brief article illustrates how to estimate financial savings from an industrial alcoholism program by using hourly wages as a proxy for the value of production lost by problem drinkers. The example chosen was a project entitled Employee Health Program, a comprehensive alcoholism referral and treatment effort serving multiple employers and unions, established in 1972 under the sponsorship of the Johns Hopkins University School of Hygiene and Public Health and the United States Department of Labor's Office of Research and Development. The goals of the project are to develop basic research on alcoholic workers and to determine the economic feasibility of establishing an outpatient treatment system to stabilize work-related behavior through a rehabilitation program. A model for return on investment measuring cost savings attributable to the program was developed and presented. It is not clear at this time whether the model has been adequately tested.

Weaver, Charles. EAPs, how they improve the bottom line. *Risk Management.* 26:22-26, July 1979.

This article describes the problems that affect work performance and provides a prototype for a risk management program. A cost-benefit analysis is given in detailed format.

Cancer

Rotkin, I. D., and Merchant, R. K. Papanicolaou smear survey of a selected industrial population. *Journal of Occupational Medicine.* 10:594-99, Oct. 1968.

The objectives of this exploratory study were to (1) determine in a population of women employed by the Pacific Telephone Company those individuals who would make up a target population for educational programs with the goal of achieving appropriate utilization of Pap smear testing; (2) determine the knowledge, attitudes, and practices of this delineated group so that a standard of comparison can be made for future studies; and (3) provide material for long-term evaluation of program effectiveness for decision makers to make changes in degree and direction of educational interventions. Approximately 8,900 questionnaires were distributed with a 63 percent rate of return (5,600 +).

From the results, the investigators were able to determine that about 90 percent of the respondents knew about the test, but an overwhelming number of the respondents clearly named their source of information as being a physician and not an educational media or school effort. Utilization was highest among married women and those who were ages 30 to 60. Almost all who learned of the test from a physician took the test, although regularity of testing was not assured in at least one-third of the sample. By far the largest interest in obtaining more information on Pap smear tests was among women in their teens and twenties who had not previously been tested. Because women of this age range constituted a large proportion of the personnel responding to the survey and a good proportion of this group named their source of information about the Pap test as someone other than a physician, the implications for promoting a cancer detection and/or education program in the work setting are that the impetus for taking the test may lie in the credibility of the source of the message as opposed to the message itself.

Hypertension

Alderman, Michael, and others. Hypertension control programs in occupational settings. In: *Proceedings of the National Conference on Health Promotion Programs in Occupational Settings.* Washington, DC: Government Printing Office, 1979.

The authors review a variety of structures for control programs conducted in the work place with varying degrees of success or failure and suggest educational strategies that appear to have the greatest promise for hypertension control in the work place. The major findings of this review suggest that positive results are short term when detection was not coupled with frequent and appropriate contact with a health care provider, social support systems, and self-monitoring of blood pressure on the part of the participant. It was emphasized that the success rate diminished without long-term followup and reinforcement. The studies reviewed did not include cost-benefit or cost-effectiveness modes of analysis, although the authors contend that the potential for savings in this area for the work place is great because hypertension is the most responsive to treatment of all the cardiovascular risk factors.

Hannon, Edward L., and Graham, J. Kenneth. A cost benefit study of a hypertension screening and treatment program at the work setting. *Inquiry.* 15:345-585, Dec. 1978.

Presented in this paper is an economic model for predicting the costs and benefits that would result from the introduction of a hypertension screening and treatment program in the work place. The expected costs and benefits are dependent on the distribution of age, sex, and blood pressure among employees; the size of the company; and the extent of an already existing medical department. If a medical department already exists, then costs of the program are incremented for personnel, size of the company, and extent of an already existing medical department.

Three types of benefits included in the study were: savings resulting from a decrease in hospital utilization and physician services, savings resulting from a decrease in disability days or absenteeism as a result of hypertension, and savings resulting from a decrease in mortality.

Various means to measure the three types of savings were described, and a discount rate of 5 percent was applied to all costs and benefits back to the beginning of the project.

The methodology included the development of a computer model to determine costs and benefits of hypertension screening over a period of one to five years. The steps for prediction are listed and explained in great detail and appear to be appropriately applied, although others are free to use a different discount rate. The authors also described the only hypertension screening and control program conducted in the work setting by Alderman and Davis and report data on program costs, frequency of hospitalization and disability, and decrease in blood pressure among members of a small self-insured union.

Several computer runs were made to test the model so that certain factors such as the size of the company and the age, sex, and blood groups of subjects in the study would reflect economies of scale. Meanwhile, the model is currently being used by the New York State Department of Health and appears promising for large randomized trials.

Stamler, Rose, and others. A hypertension control program based on the workplace. *Journal of Occupational Medicine.* 20:618-25, Sept. 1978.

In several large Chicago companies and institutions, work-place screening of 7,151 persons yielded 833 suspected hypertensive persons. Of these, 91 percent attended a follow-up verification visit, where high diastolic pressure was confirmed for 513 persons. One-half of these persons were referred to their physicians for treatment, and one-half were randomly assigned to be treated directly by the Chicago Center of the Hypertension Detection and Follow-up Program (HDFP) in a step-wise pharmacologic regimen to normalize diastolic pressure.

Of the 257 persons assigned to program treatment, 94 percent accepted such treatment, and over 90 percent of these persons still living in the community were active participants one year later. Average diastolic pressure of these active participants was 83.1 mm Hg at one year, compared with 102.6 mm Hg at the first screening and 98.8 mm Hg at the second confirmatory screening.

A strenuous effort has been made to reduce or eliminate obstacles to treatment, including lack of understanding of the need for long-term therapy, cost barriers, and barriers of inconvenience of treatment. The medical team conducting the program combined physicians with nonphysician therapists and health counselors plus outreach staff to maximize program adherence. Preliminary experiences in the Chicago Center of the HDFP give encouraging evidence that the work place is a useful base for successful hypertension control efforts.

Nutrition and Weight Control

Foreyt, John P., and others. Weight control and nutrition education programs in occupational settings. In: *Proceedings of the National Conference on Health Promotion Programs in Occupational Settings.* Washington, DC: Government Printing Office, 1979.

The emphasis in this paper is on promoting the control of eating behaviors among obese individuals who are in need of learning how to best adhere to a recommended diet for weight reduction. Studies indicating mild success utilizing behavioral techniques were reviewed; however, it was pointed out that there are currently few weight control and/or nutrition education programs that are ongoing. Those exceptions, including the first rigorously controlled study examining the experience of members of the United Store Workers Union who work at Gimbel's Department Store in New York City, are summarized. A detailed program description of behavioral techniques used at Gold King Oil Company is given, along with a presentation of positive research results obtained using a simple, uncontrolled research design on a small population. Data on the cost-effectiveness of such programs in the occupational setting was not found to be available at the time.

Physical Fitness

Bjurstron, Larry A., and Alexiou, Nicholas G. A program of heart disease intervention for public employees. *Journal of Occupational Medicine.* 20:521-31, Aug. 1978.

To apply existing knowledge of the epidemiological precursors of cardiovascular disease and therein modify risk factors associated with its ubiquitous mortality and morbidity, a behavior modification program was implemented for characteristically sedentary state employees. Available to employees regardless of age, sex, salary, or health status, the program was supported by federal, state, and employee contributions. A formal, 15-week primary intervention consisting of a progressive physical conditioning program (one hour per day, three days per week) was complemented by eight one-hour seminars. An ongoing secondary intervention program reinforced previously incorporated life-style modifications and provided opportunity for further life-style modification. The five-year experience involving 847 employees resulted in favorable modifications in risk factors, amelioration of health problems, and reductions in employee absenteeism. Similar programs should be implemented to facilitate self-health principles and practices and encourage modifications of self-imposed risks.

Haskell, William L., and Blair, Steven N. The physical activity component of health promotion programs in occupational settings. In: *Proceedings of the National Conference on Health Promotion Programs in Occupational Settings.* Washington, DC: Government Printing Office, 1978.

The authors present scientific evidence for the health and job-related benefits of increased physical activity. They also describe factors associated with motivating adults to engage in and maintain physical activity, and they describe how exercise programs are implemented in the industrial setting.

In the section on exercise and job performance, a measure of the relative physiologic stress of a given physical task was expressed as the Physical Working Capacity-Metabolic Unit (or the energy expended at rest). It appears that this measure might allow for the quantification of physical activity beyond the usual output of calories, which is not necessarily uniform across persons for the same task. It is not clear whether this measure has been validated in the work place.

Several studies which used self-reporting techniques to indicate positive changes in job productivity as a result of adherence to an exercise program are summarized, but there are no available studies that actually measure productivity itself as an outcome of increased physical activity. Most studies measuring changes in absenteeism have selection biases associated with them. Major findings were reported from studies by Heinzelmann, Bagley, and others of factors influencing recruitment of adults and their adherence to a supervised education program at NASA headquarters. Many recruitment factors were related to motivations other than for improvement of health risks. Adherence factors were related to the usual access to facilities and availability of time problems and the need for influencing persons who are important to the persons making up the target group(s) for physical exercise. Several excellent recommendations as to the appropriate components and strategies of successful employee exercise programs were made at the end of the article.

Heinzelmann, Fred, and Durbeck, Donald. *Personal Benefits of a Health Evaluation and Enhancement Program.* Heart Disease and Stroke Control Program, Regional Medical Programs, Health Service and Mental Health Administration. Mimeographed paper, 1976.

A study was made of the benefits reported by participants in a health evaluation and enhancement program dealing with physical activity. The program was conducted among employees at NASA headquarters in Washington, DC. Program benefits were identified and defined in regard to three major areas: program effects on work, program effects on health, and program effects on habits and behavior. A strong, positive, and consistent relationship was found between reported benefits in each of these areas and measures of improvement in cardiovascular functioning based on treadmill performance. Significant differences in these measures of improvement were also found between participants who reported program benefits and those persons who did not. These findings provide a meaningful profile of the pattern of benefits generated by this kind of health program.

The Perrier Study: Fitness in America. New York City: Great Waters of France, Inc., Jan. 1979.

Great Waters of France, Inc. commissioned Lou Harris and Associates to conduct a survey designed to examine in detail the knowledge, attitudes, and behavior of Americans toward physical fitness, exercise, and the relationship between preventive medicine and physical fitness. The survey included a representative sample of 1,500 persons aged 18 and over and a telephone sample of 180 runners. Based on this sample, the researchers projected that 90 million adults or 59 percent of Americans are participating in some form of physical activity. Data was presented on key perceptions about physical activity, activity levels, smoking, nutritional habits, sleep habits, and barriers to participation in physical activity. Such data would be of interest to practitioners who are interested in developing fitness programs for specific target populations.

Risk Assessment

Geotz, Axel A., and others. Health risk appraisal: the estimation of risk. In: *Proceedings of the National Conference on Health Promotion Programs in Occupational Settings.* Washington, DC: Government Printing Office, 1979.

The essence of this paper is that, at the present time, it is difficult, if not impossible, to extrapolate risk assessment to the individual when most risk assessment procedures apply to populations. At best, risk appraisal estimates the probability for mortality or morbidity resulting from particular diseases and cannot be thought of as a diagnosis.

Correspondingly, a risk estimation depends on a data base more extensive than the usual medical history and requires that a huge data base be gathered and predicted over decades, if necessary. In addition, use of risk estimations to educate individuals about their own risk in order to change behaviors directed at reduction of risk is still somewhat tenuous. The assumptions for changing the incidence of a disease process for which there are known risk indicators by altering the prevalence of these risk indicators in a defined population have not been fully tested. The point was illustrated in the case of the Stanford Heart Disease Prevention program, which reduced the prevalence of two specific risk indicators, namely, smoking and cholesterol levels. However, whether the current risk of stroke and myocardial infarction has been reduced is unknown. The North Korelia project in Finland and the Multiple Risk Factor Intervention Trial studies may yield some information on the testing of two versions of the hypothesis (full benefit versus partial benefit assumptions).

Another practical problem is the impreciseness of changing the prevalence of certain behaviors so as to influence risk in a specific population when the risk factors are not yet well defined. Past epidemiologic studies used univariate and bivariate methods of analysis when using multivariate techniques for testing effects measured separately, in combination, or interacting with one another might have yielded better results. Other methodological limitations include noncomparability of data across studies for the same risk factors, use of estimates for risk factors, and inability to predict an individual's fate with respect to a specific disease when so-called known risk factors appear to be present in an individual. There are multiple outcome possibilities depending on generic background, social support systems, psychological outlook, and various environmental influences yet untested.

Despite these methodological problems, the author provides some useful guidelines for estimating risk factors and a formula following Robbins and Petrakis's general procedure for translating relative risk values into risk factors. The problem of risk estimation and mental illness was covered with the caveat that there appears to be no information in the literature at this time to support estimation of an individual's risk for mental illness.

The prospect for improvement of risk estimation is good provided that health appraisal instruments are applied to large populations over long periods in prospective studies to gather large numbers of variables related to utilization, morbidity, and mortality outcomes, which can be arranged in large matrices and investigated through the use of appropriate analytic techniques. This prospect could be dimmed by the fact that such work requires a large amount of time, money, and personnel, although the potential payoff for predictability based on risk estimation could be high indeed.

Screening

Breslow, M. D., and Somers, Anne R. The lifetime health-monitoring program. *New England Journal of Medicine.* 296:601-608, Mar. 17, 1977.

Breslow and Somers question the efficacy of the annual physical exam and multiphasic screening and of broad health education programs in the prevention of chronic, noninfectious diseases. The authors cite the rationale behind such programs as being ill-defined and the program design and promotion fraught with "nonspecific goals and insufficient data." Breslow and Somers advocate that programs be based on major risk factors for specific populations. Questions of relevance and cost-effectiveness should be related to each group at risk for each problem.

Described is a package known as the Lifetime Health-Monitoring Program, which prescribes specific goals and professional services throughout the life span (prenatal through old age). This developmental approach reflects changing life-styles, health needs, and problems, and consequently, health goals attributed to the ten periods of life that were identified as being critical markers of such changes.

The authors present national per capita cost estimates on a fee-for-service basis for implementing such a program and call for insurance coverage and more incentives for instituting such a monitoring system. The authors hasten to note that their proposal for a lifetime health monitoring program awaits studies to test its effectiveness and cost-benefit, although their initial assumption is that instituting their program would save costs over the long-term because preventive medicine (at the secondary level) costs less than curative medicine.

Smoking Cessation

Danaher, Brian S. Smoking cessation in occupational settings: state of the art report. In: *Proceedings of the National Conference on Health Promotion Programs in Occupational Settings.* Washington, DC: Government Printing Office, 1979.

The trends of a variety of smoking cessation programs are reviewed. The magnitude of the time involved in the various efforts was questioned: the recidivism rate for one-half of the participants was high, especially in the first five weeks of a smoking cessation program. However, some hopeful behavioral research findings indicated that aversive techniques were useful but had some physiologic drawbacks. Some exemplary industrial programs using strong research designs (Ford Motor Company) and/or innovative techniques such as cash incentives (Dow Chemical, Texas Operating Division) and smoking prohibitions (Johns-Manville) are described in detail. Six recommendations are made for developing a more comprehensive approach toward smoking cessation conducted in the work place. This includes consideration of media, use of incentives, behavioral smoking control programs, self-help techniques, long-term evaluation studies, measurement of recruiting plans, and improved interaction among behavioral scientists, medical directors, and union and management leaders who are interested in smoking cessation programs conducted in the work place.

Stress Management

Peters, Raunne K., and others. Daily relaxation response breaks in a working population. II. Effects on blood pressure. *American Journal of Public Health.* 67:954-59, Oct. 1977.

A "true" experiment was conducted at the corporate office of the Converse Rubber Company to investigate the effects of daily relaxation breaks on workers' self-reported measures of health, performance, and well-being. Five variables were measured: symptoms, illness, performance, sociability-satisfaction, happiness-unhappiness. All of these variables are components of stress according to the authors' definition. The study involved 194 persons randomized into four groups. One group received instructions in a relaxation technique, one group was told to sit quietly twice per day, and two groups acted as controls. One control group consisted of nonvolunteers, and the other three groups involved volunteers. An analysis of variance was performed and yielded significant enough differences among the groups' behavioral responses and blood pressure readings to suggest that the "relaxation" instruction made an appreciable difference for the short period that the experiment was conducted.

Methodological difficulties were apparent but were addressed. It appears that a longitudinal study would have helped to demonstrate whether the effects might have been sustained over time. Certainly, more programs with appropriate evaluation designs associated with them would go far in helping advance health promotion programs in business settings. Though no cost factors were analyzed, it was pointed out that the relaxation response training involved a minimum investment of time and personnel to achieve the desired results in comparison with other programs of stress control that some employers have purchased.

Schwartz, Gary E. Stress management in occupational settings. In: *Proceedings of the National Conference on Health Promotion Programs in Occupational Settings.* Washington, DC: Government Printing Office, 1979.

This reviewer did not assume that the reader was thoroughly conversant with the field of stress management in occupational settings and started with background concepts. Schwartz defines three different types of stress and the sources from which they emanate. He emphasizes using a conceptual framework (provided in an appendix) that used an integrated psychosocial-biological approach toward stress and stress management. Sources for one type of stress would come from the work place and are job related. Techniques for stress management were listed, and their goals and procedures were described. They included assertiveness training, somatic stress management emphasizing alternating tension and relaxation of basic muscle groups, cognitive approaches, biofeedback, the "inoculation" approach used primarily for control of pain, and Benson's "relaxation" response procedures, which combine several techniques. It was generally acknowledged that a combination of procedures is probably the most effective because of the differing kinds and sources of stress and the interaction of other variables, both endogenous and exogenous, to the individual worker.

Only a few studies on the effectiveness of stress management in occupational settings were reviewed, because there was only one published that had an experimental design—Peters, Benson, and others with Converse Rubber Company. A second unpublished study was conducted by Manusco and had excellent results in the reduction of stress symptoms such as headaches. Results could not be wholly attributable to the stress management program for lack of a control group; however, Manusco did perform a true cost-benefit analysis and found that a substantial savings was accrued (ratio of 1:5.52) with the reduction of symptoms. Schwartz warns that such a ratio was overly optimistic as a result of the tentativeness of the figures.

The Emotional Health Program available to employees at Equitable Life Assurance Company of America was described. This program employs four full-time staff members, is part of the regular employees' health service, and is conducted free of charge on company time.

Recommendations for the future of stress management in the work place included:

- Incorporate stress management programs into the work place on an experimental basis to combine clinical variables with work-related variables
- Include evaluation designs that investigate long-term outcomes as well as short-term outcomes and combine clinical research with cost-effectiveness studies
- Recognize that because sources of stress include the work environment, one of the most cost-effective means of management might be to change elements of the work setting to match the needs of workers and to provide a balance between organizational requirements and employees' capacity to meet them
- Establish funds for predoctoral and postdoctoral fellowship to encourage more psychologists and other social scientists to enter the stress management field and to develop techniques for solid research and development projects in occupational settings

Additional Readings

American Hospital Association, Center for Health Promotion. *Health: What They Know, What They Do, What They Want. A National Survey of Consumers and Businesses.* Chicago: AHA, 1978.

Bauer, Katherine. *Improving the Choices for Health: Lifestyle Change and Health Education.* San Francisco: National Center for Health Education, 1980.

Cunningham, Robert M. *Wellness at Work: A Report on Health and Fitness Programs for Employees of Business and Industry.* Chicago: Blue Cross Association, 1982.

Egdahl, Richard H., and Chapman Walsh, Diana. *Springer Series on Industry*

and Health Care. New York City: Springer-Verlag, 1977-78.
- *Payer, Provider, Consumer: Industry Confronts Health Care Costs*
- *A Business Perspective on Industry and Health Care*
- *Background Papers on Industry's Changing Role in Health Care Delivery*
- *Health Services and Health Hazards: The Employee's Need to Know*
- *Industry and HMOs: A Natural Alliance*
- *Containing Health Benefit Costs: The Self Insurance Option*
- *Industry's Voice in Health Policy*
- *Women, Work and Health: Challenges to Corporate Policy*
- *Mental Wellness Programs for Employees*

Health promotion: a special issue. *Hospitals.* 53:19, Oct. 1, 1979.

Healthy People: The Surgeon General's Report on Health Promotion and Disease Prevention. Washington, DC: United States Public Health Service Office of the Surgeon General, 1979.

Hospitals and the marketplace: a special issue. *Hospitals.* 55:22, Nov. 16, 1981.

Interstudy: National Chamber Foundation. *A National Health Care Strategy.* Washington, DC: Interstudy: National Chamber Foundation. (This encompasses five reports on business involvement with health.)
- *How Business Can Promote Good Health for Employees and Their Families*
- *How Business Interacts with the Health Care System*
- *How Business Can Use Special Techniques to Control Health Care Costs*
- *How Business Can Stimulate a Competitive Health Care System*
- *How Business Can Improve Health Planning and Regulations*

Kotler, Philip. *Marketing for Non-Profit Organizations.* Englewood Cliffs, NJ: Prentice-Hall, Inc., 1975.

Minnesota Hospital Association, compiler. *The Changing Role of the Hospital: Options for the Future.* Chicago: American Hospital Association, 1980. (Catalog no. 127186).

Montana, Patrick J., editor. *Marketing in Non-Profit Organizations.* New York City: American Management Association, 1978.

Parkinson, Rebecca. *Health Promotion in the Workplace: Guidelines for Implementation and Evaluation*. Palo Alto, CA: Mayfield Publishing Co., 1982.

Rogers, Everett M. *Communication of Innovations*. New York City: Free Press, 1971.

Rubright, Robert, and MacDonald, Dave. *Marketing Health and Human Services*. Rockville, MD: Aspen Systems Corporation, 1981.

Sarason, Seymour B. *The Creation of Settings and Future Societies*. San Francisco: Jossey-Bass, Inc., 1972.

Resource Publications

Employee Health and Fitness. American Health Consultants, Inc., 67 Peachtree Park Drive, NE, Atlanta, GA 30309.

This publication, issued monthly, serves as a digest of the latest studies and experiences of employee health programs. It includes practical suggestions for program implementation from experts in the field as well as information about available program resources.

PROmoting Health. American Hospital Association, 840 N. Lake Shore Dr., Chicago, IL 60611.

Published bimonthly, this publication provides useful information and innovative ideas drawn from actual hospital experiences in the implementation of health promotion activities in hospitals. Also featured are regular articles on current issues in health promotion and a column listing current available resources.